THE NEW
HEALING
YOURSELF

Natural Remedies for Adults and Children

Also by Joy Gardner

Color and Crystals, A Journey Through the Chakras (Crossing Press)
Healing Yourself During Pregnancy (Crossing Press)
A Difficult Decision: A Compassionate Book About Abortion (Crossing Press)
The Book of Guidance (Healing Yourself Press)

THE NEW
HEALING
YOURSELF

Natural Remedies for Adults and Children

BY JOY GARDNER

The Crossing Press
Freedom, California 95019

Note to the Reader

The various treatments and suggestions made in this book, although based on information that the author has gathered from the personal experiences of a number of individuals, has neither been tested on a broad sample of individuals nor been scientifically established. Therefore, neither the author nor the publisher take responsibility for any ill effects which may be produced as a result of following any suggestions given in this book. The reader does so at his or her own risk. The author and publisher wish to stress that the suggestions offered are based on the assumption that the condition in question has been correctly diagnosed.

Copyright ©1989 Joy Gardner
Editor: Andrea Chesman
Text illustrations:
    Colored lamp & charging water, Kelly Van Dolen
    Herbs, Mimi Kamp
    Human figures, Mary Phelan
    Others, Dasa Hoffman
Cover illustration: Peter Bartczak
Cover design: Betsy Bayley
Printed in the U.S.A.

Library of Congress Cataloging-in-Publication Data

Gardner, Joy.
    The new healing yourself: natural remedies for adults and children / by Joy Gardner.
        p. cm.
    Rev. ed. of: Healing yourself. 7th rev. ed. c1982.
    Bibliography: p.
    Includes index.
    ISBN 0-89594-355-7: $26.95 (est.).—ISBN 0-89594-354-9 (pbk.)
    1. Self-care, Health. 2. Herbs--Therapeutic use. 3. Vitamin therapy. I. Gardner, Joy. Healing yourself. II. Title. RA776.95.G37 1989
    613—dc19
                                                                          88-36923
                                                                              CIP

Contents

Preface

In 1972 I compiled a little yellow booklet entitled *Healing Yourself*. It was published by the Country Doctor Clinic in Seattle as a way of encouraging patients to take responsibility for their own health and as an introduction to preventive medicine. When I left Seattle, I continued to publish the booklet myself, until 1986, when the publishing was taken over by The Crossing Press. *Healing Yourself* proved so useful it sold over 100,000 copies.

Healing Yourself was based on experience—my own and those who were willing to share their knowledge with me. Every remedy I heard of was written on an index card, to be followed by all the examples I could gather of people who tried that remedy and the results they achieved.

No remedy was ever too strange for me. My main question was, "Does it really *work*?" And then, "Will it work again? And again?"

When I first began to learn about natural healing in 1966, I learned about natural home remedies empirically, through experimentation. At first I lived on a commune in the country, where I helped find natural remedies for the various ailments of 80 people living on 200 acres of land. I learned by apprenticing with herbalists and teachers of all sorts, by reading voraciously, and by experimenting on myself and on willing friends and family. I learned by listening to anybody who would share their healing experiences: American Indians, Italian farmers, people from the Deep South, and the ladies at the laundromat. Then I worked at the Country Doctor Clinic in Seattle as a paramedic and as a herbal and nutritional consultant, and I did careful follow-up on all my clients.

Presently I work as a holistic healer and counselor in private practice in Santa Cruz, using visualization, hypnosis, emotional release, color and crystal therapy, toning, death and loss counseling, and even past-life regressions. Herbalism and nutrition continue to be an essential part of my practice. All of these healing arts will be taught by myself and others at the Santa Cruz Center of Health and Spirituality, where the emphasis will be on healing yourself, while learning to heal others. (For more information, write Healing Yourself, P.O. Box 3414, Santa Cruz, CA 95063.)

When the original *Healing Yourself* was published, I encouraged my readers to send me their favorite home remedies. I became the happy recipient of a constant stream of mail from grateful readers, including many herbalists, naturopaths, chiropractors, doctors, and nurses. So, when I decided to revise *Healing Yourself* (in 1980), I sent out long questionnaires to 100 people who had written to me.

To my amazement, about 75 dedicated and generous souls answered my questionnaire. In this way, I accumulated a contemporary analysis of natural healing as it is being practiced in North America (and elsewhere).

My first project was to compile the vast number of remedies that I had accumulated on pregnancy and childbirth. So many midwives answered my questionnaire that I was able to assemble a whole book, *Healing Yourself During Pregnancy*, which was published by The Crossing Press in 1987. The rest of the material has found its way into this edition.

I am grateful to the generous people who shared their knowledge, time, and energy: Cynthia Alexander; Shari Basom; Annamae Boutin, with La Leche League International; Sherry Gewin Brandon; Evie Brigance; Armand Ian Brint; Mimi Camp, herbalist and botanist; Anneke Campbell; Jim Campbell, M.D.; Tree Campbell, R.N.; Dave Carroll; Julie Chapman; Pip and Linda Cole, herbalists; Debbie and Herb Cox; Teresa Daffron, herbalist; Carolyn de Marco, M.D.; Isa Devora; Randy and Sandy Dorn; Claire Douglas; Carol Dunning; Meta Earthling; Fallah; Emily Finley; Laeh Maggie Garfield, author, who provided information on the underlying causes of various diseases; Elton Golden, author; James and Mindy Green, herbalists; Dan Hardt, N.D.; Mauris Harla; Monique Harrington; Lura Hirsch; Kathy Hubinet, R.N.; Hermina Hughes; Margaret Hunt; Helen Jacobs, herbalist; Kathy Karjala, nutritionist; Kathryn, R.N., from The Farm in Tennessee; Harvey A. Kryger, D.D.S., M.D.; Marc Lappe; Mary Louise Lau; Liz Lipski, nutritionist; Tina Long; Mahara, herbalist; Lisa Marsh, R.N.; Michael and Donna Marsh; Meredith and Ladd Martin; Meghan McComisky; Kathleen Harrington Meltzer, herbalist; Mrs. Judy Murray, herbalist; Norma Myers, herbalist; Faith Parker; Jo Patrick; Ray Peat, Ph.D., nutritionist; Joe Pizzorno, N.D.; Nancy Portnoy; Esther Post; Esther Rome, with Boston Women's Health Book Collective; Ellen Ruell; Sarsthi, herbalist; Afeni Shakur; Norma and Charles Shelan; Singing Tree, herbalist; Joyce Smulkis; John Joseph Snively, dentist; Elizabeth Sommers; Elizabeth Stark; Tamara; Ms. Tierney; Mrs. Dena Tremblay; Marj Watkins, herbalist; Susun Weed, author; Kay Weiss, author; Carol Wertheimer; Lasky Wilson; Laurie Wilson; Elaine Zablocki; Louise Zenev, R.N.

Also, the following books have contributed greatly to the sections on when to see a medical worker: *Healthwise Handbook* by Toni Roberts Beard, Kathleen McIntosh Tinker, and Donald W. Kemper; and *Take Care of Yourself* by Donald Vickery, M.D., and James F. Fries, M.D. Louise Hay's excellent book, *Heal Your Body, The Mental Causes for Physical Illness and the Metaphysical Way to Overcome Them*, was helpful in determining the underlying causes of various illnesses.

And finally, I wish to thank Elaine and John Gill, my publishers, whose faith in the importance of this book gave me the impetus to keep on keeping on, and Andrea Chesman, my editor, who midwifed *The New Healing Yourself* into reality.

Healing Yourself has been in existence since 1972. It has continued to grow and change and improve partly because readers have been so responsive. If you choose to try these remedies, and if you experience any unpleasant side effects, please notify me (Healing Yourself, P.O. Box 3414, Santa Cruz, CA 95063) so that in future editions of this book, I can continue to upgrade the information.

And now I hope you will join me in celebrating *The New Healing Yourself*. May you be in good health and good spirit. May you use this book well, and may it be of great service to you and your family.

Chapter 1

Health and Natural Healing

I believe that the health of our bodies is inseparable from the health of our minds, emotions, and spirits. In this book I emphasize how to use nontoxic, noninvasive remedies to heal our bodies, but I believe that physical ailments tend to have underlying emotional causes. When we become aware of the reasons for our illnesses (including stress, tension, overwork, and poor nutrition), we become better able to heal the whole person.

Included in the descriptions of most of the illnesses covered in this book are comments on the probable underlying causes of these diseases. The body speaks a language of its own and, when you learn to read that language, it will give you insight into both the cause and the cure of the disease.

This language of the body is often reflected in the folk wisdom found in the idiomatic expressions which have become an unconscious part of our vocabulary. For example, a woman may call her husband a "pain in the neck," but when she wakes up with a crick in her neck, she's more likely to explain it away by thinking that she slept in an awkward position. Another idiomatic expression: "She was green with envy." The color of bile is green, and emotions such as envy, jealousy, and anger can cause the release of excessive amounts of bile, which may affect a person's facial color.

Yet another aspect of body language relates to the right and left sides. An injury or illness that is predominantly on the left side tends to relate to problems with women (including one's mother). An injury or illness predominantly on the right side indicates possible trouble with men (including one's father) or with institutions (school, government, work).

Even so-called accidents are often outward expressions of repressed anger felt toward others. For example, insurance statistics show that people who are experiencing a divorce or separation are much more likely to be involved in automobile accidents. If we can find safe ways of expressing our hurt and anger, we'll be less likely to take it out on ourselves (or on our loved ones). Some good outlets are punching pillows, working out with a punching bag, chopping wood, and beating a mattress with a tennis racket or a rubber hose. It helps to consciously think about the people or situations that have made you angry and to vent your emotions while you perform these activities.

When you are reading about your problem in this book, consider the possible underlying cause of that ailment. You may want to discuss the underlying cause with a friend or a therapist, and it may lead to explorations that will catalyze inner growth for you. If the suggested cause does not apply to you, disregard it. If you would like to have an affirmation (a positive statement that you can repeat to yourself to help change your attitude) about a particular illness, consult Louise Hay's book, *Heal Your Body, The Mental Causes for Physical Illness and the Metaphysical Way to Overcome Them.*

Perhaps the most esoteric underlying cause of disease relates to past lives. In fact, I have found that most serious diseases that began in early childhood or at birth can be traced back to past lives.

I urge you to be open-minded. When I wrote the first edition of *Healing Yourself* in 1972, most people laughed at the idea that herbs or vitamins could heal anything. I suggest that you take an empirical approach. Try it. If it works, use it. You may say, "It's all in the mind." You may be right. If that's the case, take advantage of the mind's power to heal.

Though the main emphasis of this book is on herbal and nutritional remedies, I have made brief forays into lesser-known territories, such as color healing and Bach Flower Remedies, which are described later.

BASIC FIRST AID KIT AND SHOPPING LIST

If you want to get started with a supply of basic home remedies, where do you begin? If you want to take a few basic remedies on a backpacking trip or keep a small box of remedies in your car, which ones would be most useful?

In an attempt to answer these questions, I've compiled three lists.

If you need to conserve space, use small containers, such as film cans (clearly labeled), for the herbs. For liquids, be sure to use small, leakproof bottles. I've found that half-ounce dropper bottles (available in drugstores) are perfect because they are almost unbreakable and definitely leakproof.

Most of the items on the list can be found in drugstores, health food stores, and wherever herbs are sold. If you cannot find a specific item, or would like to do your shopping through the mail, consult the Resources section in the back of this book.

Essential Items

Rescue Remedy
Comfrey ointment
Calendula cerate or salve
Arnica tablets
Cayenne
Cinnamon
Slippery elm powder
Golden seal powder
Echinacea powder
Valerian root powder
Tiger Balm
Size 00 gelatin caps
Band-aids

Highly Desirable Items

Vitamin C powder
Calms Forte
White oak bark
Gauze
Adhesive
Hydrogen peroxide
Small scissors
Cotton swabs
Castor oil
Witch hazel
Green soap

Useful Items

Coltsfoot
Peppermint
Mullein
Ephedra
Elder flowers
Garden sage
Corn silk
Essential Balm
Oil of bitter orange
Honey

PREPARATION OF REMEDIES

The remedies given in this book are usually given as recipes for teas. I am assuming that you will be using dried herbs.

To make a tea of leaves and flowers of delicate texture, place a measured amount of the herb in a nonaluminum container (ceramic, glass, or enamel). Boil water in a nonaluminum container and pour the appropriate amount of boiling water over the herbs. Cover the container for 5 to 15 minutes to allow the herbs to steep. Unless otherwise recommended, it is usually not necessary to strain an herbal tea as the leaves settle to the bottom of the pot after about 10 minutes of steeping.

To prepare a tea of tough, thick leaves (such as comfrey or mullein), bring the water to a boil, reduce the heat to a gentle rolling boil (simmer), and add the leaves to cook gently for 10 minutes. This method is also good for roots that have been granulated (chopped fine), but since roots are denser, more time is needed to extract their healing powers. Whole roots or root pieces should be added to the simmering water and cooked for 20 minutes.

When fresh herbs are used, measure twice as much as the recipe calls for, because dehydration (drying) takes out about half the weight and bulk. Fresh herbs are always preferable to dried herbs because they contain more of the essential oils and other healing properties.

Some teas, such as Lung Tea, which is used to treat asthma and chest congestion, require mixing several different herbs together. If you prepare this tea or any other complex tea frequently, you can save a lot of time by premixing all the herbs. If the recipe calls for 1 tablespoon each of several different herbs, mix together 1 cup each of the herbs. Then measure out as many tablespoons of the mix as you would have measured out for the individual herbs (i.e., if a recipe calls for 1 tablespoon of 6 different herbs, measure out 6 tablespoons of the premixed herbs for the same strength tea).

Some herbs, such as valerian, have an unpleasant taste; others, such as slippery elm, have a peculiar texture. The best way to take these herbs is in gelatin capsules that you make yourself. Empty gelatin capsules are available in most drugstores and health food stores. Buy the size marked 00; these each hold about 1/4 teaspoon of powdered herb. For best results, swallow the capsule with warm water or tea to help it dissolve. Powdered herbs are easily absorbed by the body, and taking herbs in gelatin capsules is often more convenient than preparing a cup of tea.

When purchasing herbs, try to find a reputable herb store. Find a place where the herbs are likely to be relatively fresh. You may have to pay a little more for high-quality herbs, but it's well worth it. After 1 year, most herbs lose their healing properties.

Ideally, try to get herbs that have been harvested from plants that grow naturally in the wild (wild-crafted). These herbs have selected their own optimum habitat, so they are likely to be richest in natural minerals and healing properties. In any case, when selecting dried herbs, look for the ones that have retained their color. Take a pinch of the herb and crush it in your hand to see if it has retained its natural odor. Take a nibble and see if it has a strong flavor (most herbs do).

The more the herb has been exposed to air—through processing and storage—the quicker it will lose its healing properties. Powdered herbs lose their potency faster than any other form, so don't try to stock up on more than you are likely to need for the year, and try to get them from a reliable source.

Always store herbs away from direct sunlight. Label your containers with the name of the herb and the year you obtained it. For best results, replace your herbs each year.

Tinctures are a convenient way to take herbs. High-quality tinctures are usually prepared from fresh herbs that have been harvested at the peak of the season and then chopped up and covered with ethyl alcohol (vodka, gin) and left in a dark place for about 2 weeks. The alcohol draws out the healing properties of the herb, and also preserves those properties—usually for several years.

Tinctures are convenient because you can carry them with you and take them any time you need them without having to boil water for tea. They vary in strength, so the dosage is usually given on the bottle. The equivalent of a cup of tea is usually about 5 drops. This can be taken directly under the tongue (where it is absorbed quickly into the bloodstream) or it can be added to water or juice.

Harvesting Herbs

Harvesting fresh herbs is a great joy. I particularly enjoy finding herbs growing in the wild and collecting them in the right season. When you've lived in one place for a while, you come to know where to go for each of your favorite herbs—if you're lucky enough to live in an area where wild things are allowed to grow and where people are allowed to gather them.

Be careful to avoid places where herbicides and toxic sprays are used. Always keep *at least* 10 feet away from roads. And do respect parks and areas where the public is asked not to pick the flowers or disturb the plants. Never pick more than two-thirds of a stand of herbs; allow enough to remain so it will reseed itself the next year. Never pick where there are only a few of a species and avoid endangered species.

Of course, you can also grow your own favorite herbs, and it's nice to have a herb garden both for medicine and for cooking.

Ideally, herbs should be gathered in the morning, just as the dew has dried. By afternoon on a hot day, the sun has sapped much of the essential strength of the herbs. Don't gather on a wet day, because the excess moisture will make it hard to dry the herbs, and this may cause mold. When gathering the leaves of herbs, try to get them before the plant flowers, because more of the healing properties are in the leaves at that time. Flowers, of course, are gathered when the plant is in full flower. Roots are best gathered in the fall, after the flowers have been shed, when the energy of the plant returns to the roots.

Leaves should not be washed (unless they are quite dirty), but roots need to be thoroughly washed (a hose will often do the trick) and often scrubbed with a soft brush.

Most herbs can be dried by tying a fistful of stems together with a string. I like to use a string that is 2 or 3 feet long. I wrap one end several times around one bunch of herbs and wrap the other end around another bunch. Then I can sling the herbs over my shoulder while I'm walking and hang them over a nail or a rafter for drying.

Herbs should be dried in a warm, dry place, away from direct light. Attics are ideal. Dehydrators are another good way to dry herbs, especially leaves such as comfrey (which tend to turn black when hung). They are also excellent for drying roots. If you don't have a dehydrator, dry the roots on a screen. Roots will dry faster if they are sliced or chopped, and the small size facilitates making small amounts of tea. It's hard to chop a dried root.

You'll know when the herb is fully dried because when you bend it, it will snap or crumble.

Herb Combinations

To the best of my knowledge, all herbs can be combined safely with other herbs and foods, with one exception. Chamomile will counter the healing properties of comfrey, so these two herbs should not be taken together.

Aluminum

Aluminum is toxic to the body. If you boil water in an aluminum pot, you will actually see light, feathery particles of aluminum in the water.

Aluminum has been found to cause gas, abdominal pain, diarrhea or constipation, hemorrhoids, itchy anus, duodenal ulcers, kidney and bladder problems, eye problems, itchy skin, extreme sensitivity to alcohol, thrombosis, and indecisiveness. It may also be implicated as a cause of cancer.

Do not boil water or cook food in aluminum. (It's not as harmful to cover food with foil.) Avoid drinking or cooking with hot tap water because many hot water heaters are made of aluminum. Cover the food in your refrigerator because the freezing element is usually made of aluminum, which dissipates over the contents of the refrigerator, giving the food a tinny taste. Avoid baking powder that contains aluminum (read the label). And also try to avoid deodorants that contain this mineral.

If you think you're suffering from aluminum poisoning, see a homeopathic doctor to obtain an antidote for aluminum.

NATURAL HEALING METHODS

Some of the healing methods used in this book may be unfamiliar to you. Here is a brief description of a few of these.

Color Healing

The concept of healing with color will be new to many people, but it is an ancient therapeutic technique that is now being revived.

Most people have felt the healing power of the sun as its penetrating rays coursed through their bodies, giving them energy and stimulating their skin. And most of us have also felt how long exposure to the sun can result in a draining of energy and sunburn.

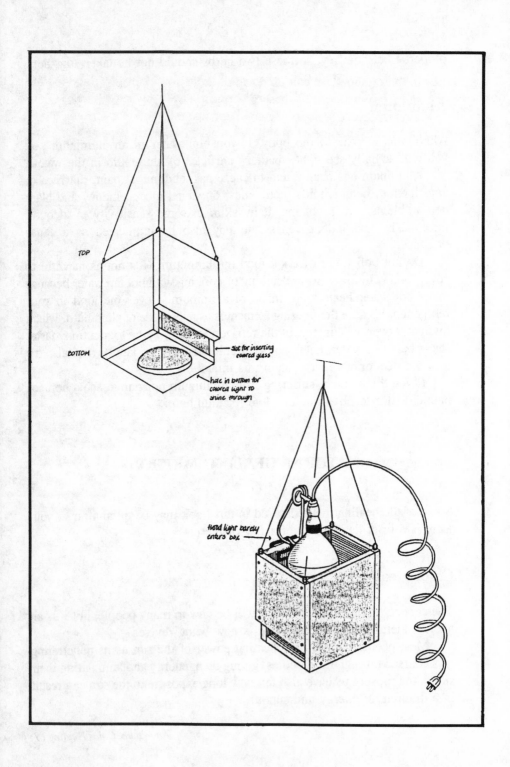

TOP

BOTTOM

Slot for inserting colored glass

hole in bottom for colored light to shine through

flood light barely enters box

Similarly, by dividing the sun's rays into its 7 component colors as they occur in the rainbow, we can use each of these colors for healing. And in some cases, an overdose of these colors can cause adverse effects.

There are many ways to use color for healing. You can introduce the color into your environment—with flowers, paintings, cloth hangings, or even by painting the room or objects in the room the desired color. (Be cautious about painting the room, because your need for a color is likely to change.) Wear clothing in the color you need. If you have a problem on a particular area of the body, wear colored clothes that cover that area (for example, wear a blue shirt for back pain).

Alternatively, you can build or buy a lamp that has colored gels (thin plastic used for theater lighting and available in theater supply stores and some paint stores) or pieces of stained glass (available at stained glass shops), through which you can shine a spotlight bulb (available in electric supply stores) to direct that color onto particular areas of the body. This is called a color bath. It should not be attempted without a complete understanding of the method.

Red light is particularly potent and should be used only for a few minutes. Usually you will not use it on your head. Red stimulates the circulation and nervous system, so it should not be used if you are nervous, agitated, or have high blood pressure. Blue is the antidote for red, and it can be used for calming any agitation. It can be used if you have received too much red. But blue is also powerful, and if you fall asleep under a blue light or lie under it for more than 30 minutes, you may feel withdrawn. A few minutes under the orange or yellow light will revive you.

You can also eat and drink colored foods and liquids. For example, red is good for the bladder and cranberry juice is excellent for bladder infections. Also, charge up and drink colored waters. The French word for water is *eau*, which is pronounced "o." So the waters are named with the suffix "o." Red water is called rubio; orange or yellow water is ambero; green water is verdo; blue water is ceruleo; purple water is purpuro; and violet water is violeo.

Water can be charged with a particular color by placing it under a colored lamp. Or by putting a piece of colored glass or gel in a sunny window with a jar of water on the windowsill in front of it, so the sun shines through the glass and reflects that color into the water. Or you can put the water in a bottle made of the appropriate colored glass. Green wine bottles, for example, can be used to charge green water.

CHARGING COLORED WATER

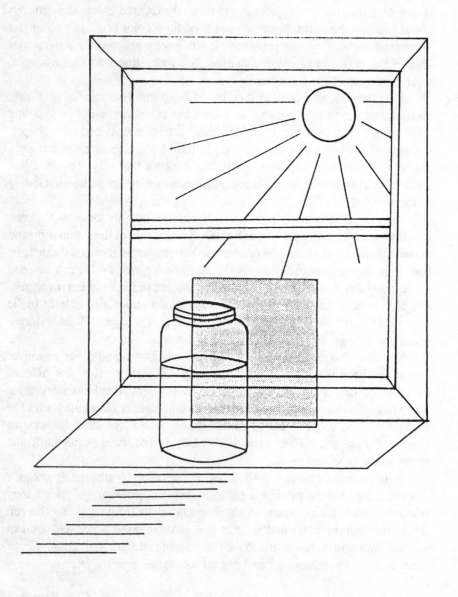

It takes 1 to 3 hours to charge colored water (the longer the stronger). Purpuro (purple water) and ceruleo (blue water) will last indefinitely, but ambero (yellow or orange water) and rubio (red water) must be kept in the refrigerator or in a cool place or else they will lose their potency in 3 or 4 days during warm weather. Even when kept cold, they must be recharged every 2 weeks.

Colored waters are used for internal problems, such as constipation and ulcers, and to aid digestion. Sometimes they are remarkably effective. The dosage will vary, but usually a few swallows are taken. A swallow can be measured as a tablespoon for an adult and as a teaspoon for a child.

The study of this form of healing is fascinating. If you would like to pursue it, see my book, *Color and Crystals* (The Crossing Press, 1988).

Healing With Stones (Crystal Healing)

As I see it, all of the colors of the rainbow appear in the electromagnetic energy that surrounds the body, which is your aura. When there is a serious physical, emotional, or spiritual imbalance, certain colors may be impure, blotchy, muddy, or entirely missing from the aura. These discolorations or omissions (which are visible to those who have inner vision) will eventually lead to physical illness.

When you use crystals and other gemstones, you allow the aura of the crystal or stone to mix with your own. Through its dominant energy, which is a particular color, it clears and brightens that color in your aura, thus removing blocks and helping you to re-establish your balance. Clear quartz crystals carry the energy of all the colors, which is why they are used for balancing the energies.

The stones can be rough or worked by humans in various ways. They can be tumbled in a rock tumbler, which is a process similar to rolling them around in a creek bed. They can be cut into various shapes to make jewel quality gemstones, the most common of which is the oval cabochon. The translucent (clear) stones can be faceted into shapes that are intended to make the stone catch the light more effectively. The tumbled or jewel quality gems are best for making tinctures and charging water, alcohol, or oil, since there are no particles to come out in the liquid. Gemstones and tumbled stones are good for smoothing over rough situations. Smooth, gem quality, and translucent stones help bring light into dark situations. On the other hand, rough stones penetrate to the depths and bring buried feelings to the surface. Rough and smooth stones can be used interchangeably if you don't happen to have exactly the right kind of stone—both are effective. When buying stones you should have a good feeling about them—that is the best guideline.

In most cases, larger stones of any particular grouping are more powerful than smaller stones. In other words, a large rose quartz is usually more powerful than a small rose quartz. Of course, a small diamond may be more powerful than a large rose quartz.

But even within a particular grouping, some small stones are unusually powerful. Deep rich colors bring greater intensity to a stone, as does a strong design. (In some cases, as with amethyst, pale colors also have a high value.) For example, the bulls-eye is inherent in the pattern of the malachite, and a small stone with a clearly defined bulls-eye is more powerful than a larger, less-defined stone.

Experiment on yourself. Begin by using the crystal energization described below. Always lie on your back with your head to the north when doing any layout to align your spine with the earth's axis and the earth's magnetic energy. Since clear quartz crystals grow naturally in veins that follow the earth's magnetic fields, and since they contain iron oxide which is a magnetic material, they are more effective when you respect their magnetic properties.

The stones can be placed over the clothing, but they are more effective when in direct contact with the skin—especially if they are small stones.

Crystal Energization. This simple practice has the extraordinary ability to pull out tension and negativity and then to recharge you with positive energy. It only takes 10 minutes and it's better than a nap. Perhaps one day it will replace coffee.

This layout requires four clear quartz, single terminated crystals (crystals that have a single point at one end and a base at the other end, as distinct from crystals that have two or more points). These crystals should be at least 1-1/2 inches long, but they don't have to be special or beautiful. In fact, if you do this on a bed, they are liable to fall off and get chipped, so don't use your favorite crystals for this layout.

Each crystal should be placed so that the terminations face outward, away from the center of your body. Place them 2 to 6 inches from your body. Lie down on a flat surface and place the crystals in these locations (see illustration):

1. Above the center of the top of your head.
2. Between and below your feet.
3. To the right of your right wrist.
4. To the left of your left wrist.

Lie in this position for about 10 minutes. Be sure no one is in the line of fire with the terminations of the crystals. Don't worry if you fall asleep.

While doing this layout, you can simultaneously place any other stones that you feel may be beneficial for you on the appropriate parts of your body.

Cleansing the Stones. Whenever you use stones for getting rid of negativity, it's a good idea to clean them. There are many elaborate methods of cleansing, but I find that the simplest is to hold them under cold running tap water for 10 to 15 seconds. Since energy follows water, the undesirable energy will wash down the drain. It is also a good idea to put your hands and wrists under cold running water.

Clear quartz crystals absorb and hold energy, so it is especially important to do this with your crystals. Hold the crystal with the termination pointing downward, toward the drain.

When you receive a new crystal, or if your crystal has been doing especially difficult work, it's a good idea to bury it in sand or dirt or put it in salt water for 1 to 3 days. Salt water can be prepared by dissolving 1 tablespoon of sea salt in 1 quart of warm water. Or you can use ocean water. Keep a container of sand or dirt for burying your stones; you can use it repeatedly, but change it periodically. If you only use it a couple times a month for special stones, you can keep the same sand, dirt, or water for 3 to 6 months. Arrange the stones so that there's at least 1 inch of space between them.

Homeopathy

This is a branch of medicine which is not widely recognized by the medical profession, despite the fact that many homeopaths are doctors. Homeopathy uses homeopathic preparations, which are derived from plant, mineral, or animal sources. These preparations are chosen according to the principle of "let like be treated by like." For example, epilepsy (a convulsive disease)

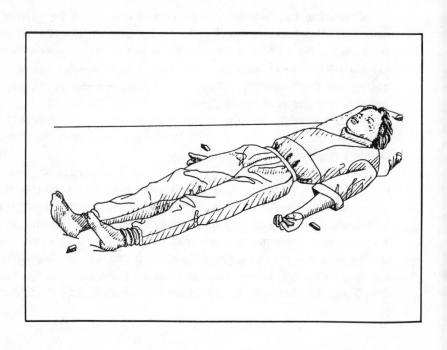

may be treated by a plant which, in large doses, produces convulsions. A minute amount of this plant is combined with a larger amount of inert material (such as alcohol), and this is then triturated or rubbed down by a machine so that the 2 substances are finely mixed. This produces a potentized remedy, which has a more powerful curative reaction in the body than a greater quantity of the original crude substance, and yet it is harmless. For example, homeopathic (or potentized) poison ivy is sometimes used to treat allergy to poison ivy. Potencies are designated by a numeral and the letter X and follow the decimal scale. The homeopathic remedies mentioned in this book can be ordered from the Standard Homeopathic Company (see Resources).

Homeopathic remedies should not be combined with any other foods, herbs, supplements, or even toothpaste within 15 minutes of taking the remedy. Also, coffee, chamomile, and strong-smelling herbs, such as eucalyptus and menthol, should be avoided on days that you take a homeopathic remedy.

Naturopathy

Naturopathy is a system of disease treatment that emphasizes assisting nature. It includes the use of nonpoisonous remedies such as herbs, vitamins, cell salts, homeopathic remedies, manipulation, electrical therapies, and hydrotherapy. A naturopathic doctor (N.D.) generally receives 4 years of education in this field, with a strong emphasis on the sciences. They are not allowed to write prescriptions for drugs. Naturopathy is legal in some states and illegal in others.

Chiropractics

Chiropractics is a system of treating disease by manipulating the vertebral column. It is based on the theory that most diseases are caused by pressure on the nerves because of faulty alignment of bones, especially the vertebrae, and that the nerves are thus prevented from transmitting to various organs of the body the neural impulses for proper functioning. A chiropractor goes to chiropractic college for approximately 4 years to learn a drugless approach to illness, which includes manipulating various parts of the spine.

Bach Flower Remedies

The Bach Flower Remedies were formulated by Edward Bach, a British doctor who, at the turn of the century, became discouraged with trying to cure physical ailments without dealing with the underlying emotional problems. Something of a mystic, he gave up his successful practice in London and moved to the countryside, where he began to induce in himself various states of emotional and physical illness. He then wandered over the hillsides, looking for flowers to bring his altered emotional states back into equilibrium. He found 38 flowers, each for a different state of mind, and developed a method of preparing tinctures from these flowers. These tinctures can be used separately or in combination, according to the needs of the individual. The Bach Flower Remedies are not a substitute for therapy or for working out real life problems; they simply bring a person into a more favorable state, from which they can better cope with their problems.

One particular combination of flower tinctures is called the Rescue Remedy because it is ideally suited for emergency situations. The Rescue Remedy is made from the flowers of star of Bethlehem (for shock), rock rose (for terror and panic), impatiens (for mental stress and tension), cherry plum (for desperation), and clematis (for the faraway feeling that often precedes fainting or loss of consciousness).

Do not attempt to make your own tea from these flowers. Like homeopathic remedies, the Bach Flower Remedies are so dilute that they are harmless; a tea could be toxic. All the remedies can be ordered through the mail (see Resources). You can order a 1-ounce bottle of Rescue Remedy, or the full set of 38 tinctures, which would enable you to make up your own combinations of remedies.

GUIDELINES FOR GOOD EATING

The I Ching (ancient Chinese book of wisdom) teaches us: Pay heed to the providing of nourishment and to what you fill your mouth with, because what you take in and how you do so will strongly influence what you give out and the effect you have.

Good nutrition is central to good health, so we can all benefit from paying full attention to what and how we eat. There's no point in learning how to heal yourself if you haven't learned how to feed yourself. By eating food in its most natural form you can take advantage of all possible vitamins and enzymes (the known ones and the undiscovered ones). By avoiding excessive eating, junk food, synthetic and processed foods, and excessive fats, you can lift a great and unnatural burden from your organs, which were never designed to handle such "foods."

We cannot be healthy if we eat food that has no vitality. Chemical fertilizers destroy the vitality of the soil, and food grown in such soil lacks some of the vital nutrients for a healthy body. So try to get organic food whenever possible.

The best way to know what you are eating is to grow it yourself, with compost and manure and mulch. Be sure you are not paying "novelty" prices for basic foods, which is what happens at many health food stores. Find out if there are any co-ops in your area. These stores usually offer high-quality food at reasonable prices.

Pay attention to how you prepare your food. If your state of mind is harmonious while you are cooking, then the food will carry that vibration of harmony.

How you eat is also important. It is a good idea to eat only when you are hungry and to stop eating when you feel satisfied (don't wait until you feel stuffed). Avoid eating when you are angry, tense, or nervous—or eat very simple foods, such as fresh juice, yogurt, and fruit. Chew your food thoroughly.

If you want to change your diet, do so gradually. Let moderation, satisfaction, and a sense of well-being be your guides.

What to Eat

At least three-quarters of your diet should consist of fruits, vegetables, whole grains, and dairy products (optional). The remaining one-quarter of your diet can then allow for personal choices.

Fruits. Fruit should be mostly fresh. Dried fruit is also acceptable.

Vegetables. Vegetables should be freshly prepared whenever possible. Wash and scrub if necessary, but try to avoid peeling and scraping, which eliminates valuable minerals. Eat your vegetables raw, or steam them in a pot with a close-fitting lid, or stew them in their own juices. Whenever water is used for cooking, save it for soups. Dried vegetables are also acceptable, but frozen or boiled vegetables lose nutrients.

Whole Grains. The best, most nutritious part of the grain is lost when you eat white flour, white rice, white cornmeal, or refined and instant cereals (rolled oats are okay). Most packaged cereals have the best part of the grains removed, and then nutrients are added artificially, along with lots of white sugar, artificial flavorings, and preservatives. Ninety-eight percent of the vitamin E is lost in the process that makes cornflakes. Seventy percent of the vitamin E is lost in rice cereal products.

Grains begin to lose their nutrients within 2 hours of being ground, and a significant proportion is lost within 2 weeks. So it's best if you can grind your own grains at home for pancakes, cereal, and bread. Or encourage your local co-op or health food store to sell fresh-ground grains.

Milk and Milk Products. These can be used in moderation, if they agree with you. Cultured milk products, such as yogurt and kefir, are the easiest for the body to assimilate. Cream and ice cream should be restricted to a minimum as they are high in saturated fat.

Other Foods. Desserts are fine as an occasional treat, and when prepared with whole grain flour and sweetened with honey, maple sugar, molasses, or brown sugar. When baking with baking powder, try to find a brand that doesn't contain aluminum.

Use salt in moderation. Try sea salt, which is higher in minerals than common table salt. Or use BioSalt, which contains all the basic cells salts in proper proportion, so that you don't get an excess of sodium, which is bad for the heart.

Try to avoid or minimize alcohol, tobacco, coffee, caffeine, soda pop, black tea, baking soda, smoked fish and other smoked meats, and black pepper.

Try to minimize red meats, and if you eat meat at all, eat mostly fish and poultry. It makes sense to eat less meat. Just from an ecological point of view, the average cow has to eat 21 pounds of protein in order to produce 1 pound of protein in the form of meat. It's possible to raise your own animals more efficiently. A cow can eat grass and other humanly inedible roughage, such as corn husks and pea vines. Animals raised at home, on land that has not been sprayed with chemicals, will produce high-quality milk, eggs, and meat.

Try to avoid meat from animals that have been injected with antibiotics and artificial estrogens to hasten their growth. Commercially raised animals live and die under depressing circumstances; their internal organs are limp and watery and barely capable of sustaining life; their eggs are pale and thin and almost tasteless.

You can obtain excellent protein from non-meat sources through combining foods with complementary amino acids. This method is explained thoroughly in *Diet for a Small Planet* by Frances Moore Lappé. She explains that proteins consist of 22 separate amino acids, 8 of which are essential amino acids that cannot be synthesized by our bodies. By the end of each day, all of these 8 essential amino acids must have been consumed and in a particular proportion, because if any one of them is in a disproportionately small amount, your body will not be able to synthesize the other amino acids into a whole protein, and so they will be used for fuel, as if they were carbohydrates.

Eggs, seafood, dairy products, meat, and poultry are whole proteins, so they need no supplementation from other foods, but small amounts of these foods make excellent supplements in themselves. Seafoods can be combined with grains, nuts, or seeds. Dairy products can be combined with grains, nuts, seeds, legumes, or potatoes. For example, mashed potatoes and milk make a good combination. Legumes (dried peas, beans, lentils) should be eaten with nuts, seeds, or grains, *and* milk (for example, a peanut butter sandwich and milk). Sunflower and sesame seeds are higher in protein than most other nuts and seeds. Sesame seeds are much more nutritious in their unhulled form, and far more digestible when ground. Cashews can be eaten alone as an excellent source of protein. Nuts and seeds are complemented by legumes, dairy products, seafood, *and* other nuts and seeds and grains. A good combination is granola containing sunflower and sesame seeds and wheat germ with milk.

NUTRITION FOR INFANTS

Breast milk is the perfect food for babies. If the infant is satisfied, mother's milk alone is adequate nourishment for at least 6 months. Before a child is 3 months old, the introduction of solids can be harmful because the solids crowd out the milk, the child nurses less, and the milk supply diminishes. Also, the early introduction of solids may set off allergic reactions since the digestive system of an infant is so immature.

When babies are old enough to sit up, they usually like to be with the family during meals. Once their teeth appear, they may begin to show an interest in food. Or there may be a sudden increase in demand to be nursed. First make sure that the baby has had enough milk, then, if there is an interest in food, introduce just 1 food at a time. Wait 5 days before introducing another. After beginning a new food, be alert for possible reactions, such as vomiting, wheezing, or rashes. If this occurs, eliminate the food for a week, then try again. If the reaction recurs 2 or 3 times, avoid the food for at least 6 months.

If there are allergies in your family, start with just 1/4 teaspoon of a new food, once or twice a day. Be especially carefully with foods that commonly produce allergic reactions, such as wheat, corn, egg whites, cow's milk, pork, fish, citrus (including orange juice), berries, nuts, onions, tomatoes, cabbage, condiments, and chocolate.

Babies do not need canned, expensive baby foods. These often contain food additives and pesticide residues. Also, most canned foods are overheated during processing. In some cases, the foods are oversweetened or oversalted.

Your own food is likely to be of higher quality (especially if it is organic), with no preservatives and no additives. Just mash it up and see if your baby wants some. A baby food grinder is useful, and you can carry it with you to restaurants. You can offer it on a spoon (baby spoons are nice), or just put a dab on the highchair tray and see if your little one takes an interest.

Once the baby is 3 months old, you can offer the following food supplements, which are high in iron and minerals. Since they take longer to digest than milk, they will also help to establish longer sleep patterns.

Apricots. Dried apricots can be covered with water and soaked overnight. You can feed the juice to the baby and eat the apricots yourself. When the baby is ready to eat foods, you can grind them in a baby grinder or puree them in a blender.

Wakame Seaweed. Put 3 inches of wakame seaweed (available in most health food stores) in a cup and pour 1 cup of boiling water over the seaweed. Soak for 20 minutes, then feed the soaking water to the baby. When the baby begins to eat solids, you can mix the seaweed with other vegetables, such as carrots, and blend or grind. Before then, mix it with your own vegetables.

Miso Soup. Bring 1 cup of water to a boil. Place 1/2 teaspoon miso (fermented soybean paste, available in health food stores) in a cup and add a little boiling water. Dissolve the miso in the water, then add the remaining water, stir, and let sit for a few minutes. Feed the broth to the baby.

For information on formulas and instructions for babies who are not breast-fed, see *Let's Have Healthy Children* by Adele Davis.

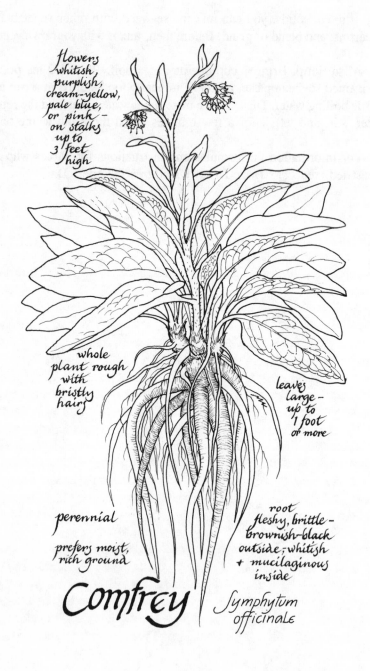

flowers
whitish,
purplish,
cream-yellow,
pale blue,
or pink –
on stalks
up to
3 feet
high

whole
plant rough
with
bristly
hairs

leaves
large –
up to
1 foot
or more

perennial

prefers moist,
rich ground

root
fleshy, brittle –
brownish-black
outside; whitish
+ mucilaginous
inside

Comfrey   Symphytum officinale

Chapter 2

Common Ailments and Treatments

This book is not meant to be a substitute for a doctor. Doctors are well trained in diagnosis, and if anything is seriously wrong with you, find a doctor, naturopath, chiropractor, or other medical worker whom you can trust. Don't fool around with self-diagnosis. Once you know what is wrong, you may benefit from this material.

We are, admittedly, our own guinea pigs. But we can be assured that most healing herbs have been a part of the human experience for thousands of years.

In this section you will find symptoms and remedies for many common complaints, ranging from aches and pains to warts. Please note that some of the remedies include comfrey, which contains minute amounts of cancer-causing substances. I discussed this with Norman Farnsworth, Ph.D., head of the Department of Pharmacology and Pharmacognosy at the University of Illinois. He tested many samples of comfrey roots and leaves and found small amounts of cancer-causing substances in most roots and in some leaves.

His personal opinion is that probably it is not harmful for an adult male or nonpregnant female to drink comfrey leaf tea 2 to 3 times a week. However, in the case of a pregnant woman, even a minute amount of a possibly harmful substance could harm the fetus. He suggests that pregnant women avoid comfrey tea entirely, although external use of comfrey in ointments and salves is all right. For children, occasional use is probably safe and comfrey salve is okay to use.

Note: Many people grow comfrey in their gardens. To dig the roots, wait until the autumn, when the energy of the plant goes into the roots. Chop off all the leaves. Then use a shovel and dig 6 to 8 inches out from the stem, in a circle, around the plant. Then you should be able to lift out a large clump of dark roots. These can be rinsed with a hose, and then brought inside for more careful cleaning. If you leave just 1 root in the ground, the plant will continue to reproduce.

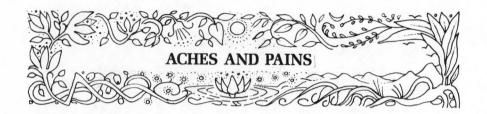

ACHES AND PAINS

Aches and pains and even accidents often occur when you are under stress—especially when you are feeling stress over a love relationship. If you feel unlovable, you are more likely to overwork or put yourself in a dangerous position. When you have been hurt by life or love, being in pain or having an "accident" gives you a good excuse to complain and even to cry.

Save yourself the trouble. When you've been hurt, go off by yourself and cry your heart out. Or find a friend whose shoulder you can cry on. Don't keep a stiff upper lip. The pain that you cover up now will go deep inside your body and reappear weeks or years later as some form of illness or "accident." Acknowledge your pain and grief. Give your emotions their rightful place.

This section will give you simple remedies for aches and pains. They should help to alleviate the muscular pain that often accompanies overwork, overexertion, tension, and strains. If you have a sprain or a more serious injury, be sure to consult a medical worker, or at least a good first aid book. For general soreness, don't forget your hot water bottle or heating pad. A good massage or sauna can be wonderfully relaxing.

External Treatments

Hot and Cold Bath or Shower. The bathtub in every home is a major contribution of modern civilization. Virtually every ache and pain will loosen its clutches while immersed in a hot bath.

But don't stop there. A cool bath will increase your circulation and enhance your sense of well-being and give you a shot of renewed energy. Allow a couple of inches of water to escape from your bath, and then add some cold water until your bath becomes tolerably cool. Continue letting out warm water and adding cold water until you reach your cold threshold.

Then sit in the cool bath briefly, emerge, and rub your body briskly with a towel.

If you haven't time for all this, you can do the same with a shower. Begin with a warm shower, and then gradually reduce the hot water. Allow the cool water to go over your back and your head (and if you're brave, the front of your body). Then reduce the hot water some more, and repeat the process. Over a period of time, you'll probably find that your tolerance for cold water increases, and you'll begin to enjoy these energizing cool baths and showers.

Hot and Cold Soak. If the pain is in a small area, it can be soaked in a basin. Soak in cold water for about 10 minutes, and then in hot water for 3 to 5 minutes. If you wish, you can continue alternating hot and cold.

Herbal Bath. We all need to be loved and pampered. When you are in pain, your body is crying out for attention. Don't be afraid to indulge yourself. This sweet-smelling bath is a wonderful way to alleviate general aches and pains, muscle cramps, tension, insomnia, and headaches—and it will even prevent the soreness and bruising that sometimes accompanies Rolfing and other deep tissue body work. Usually 25 minutes is long enough to stay in this bath, unless you want to sleep in the tub.

Bring 4 cups water to a boil, remove from the heat, and add 2/3 cup linden flowers and 1/3 cup rosemary leaves. Cover the pot and steep for 10 minutes. Strain and add to the bath water.

Epsom Salts in the Bath. Epsom salts are a form of magnesium, which is very soothing to tense muscles. Run hot water in the tub and add about 1 cup of salts. When they dissolve, adjust the temperature and run a normal bath, soaking as long as you like.

Thermophore. This is a moist heat pack that looks like a heating pad, but it is far more penetrating for aching muscles, bones, and ligaments. It is excellent for back and neck problems, arthritis, rheumatism, sciatica, stomachaches, and other aches, pains, and muscular soreness. This electric unit works by drawing moisture from the air, which means that you'll place a dry pad on your skin, and when you remove it 30 minutes later, your skin will be wet. It gives relief by easing tension through penetrating warmth. Relief may short or long-lasting.

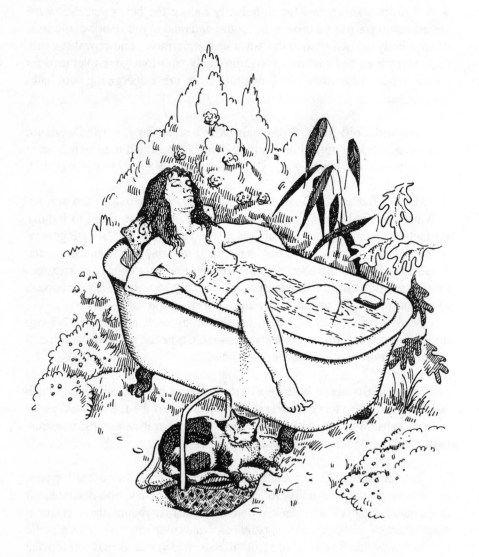

This wonderful device can be applied 2 to 3 times daily at intervals of 6 to 8 hours. Of course, the thermophore cannot be expected to cure structural problems, so if you are having chronic pain, be sure to seek help.

Thermophores come in 3 sizes. The standard size (13 inches by 27 inches) covers your whole back. The medium size (13 inches by 13 inches) is especially good for children and for small areas of the body. The petite size is used for relief of minor pain in small body areas such as the neck, throat, and sinuses.

Unfortunately, the cost of this wonderful device is a bit high, but anyone with chronic pain can hardly afford to be without one. Special instructions are provided with the thermophore and should be followed carefully. Thermophores are available from the Battle Creek Equipment Company (see Resources).

Color. The color blue is calming, soothing, and anti-inflammatory, so it is particularly soothing. Since red is stimulating and irritating, it should be avoided.

Tiger Balm. This salve is effective when there is pain in a small area. It brings intense heat within 5 to 10 minutes after applying. It stimulates circulation and breaks up congestion. Tiger Balm is made from strong aromatic oils of camphor, menthol, peppermint, clove, and cajeput. (Cajeput is an oil from the East Indies that contains methyl salicylate, which is anti-inflammatory.) There are 2 kinds of Tiger Balm: red and white. The red is considerably hotter than the white and works well on the back, chest, and extremities. The milder white is best for the face and for children. Keep Tiger Balm out of the reach of children, because camphor is poisonous when taken internally. Keep away from eyes and mucous membranes, because it causes a burning sensation. (To avoid accidentally rubbing my eyes with a finger that has Tiger Balm on it, I use the fourth or fifth finger of my left hand to apply it.)

Tiger Balm is made in China and sold in many stores where Chinese items are found, as well as many herb and health food stores. It comes in small and large vials.

White Flower Oil. This oil is also from China; it is similar to Tiger Balm, but more penetrating. Since it is an oil rather than a salve, it can be used easily over a large area, though it works well in small areas. White

Flower Oil is made with strong aromatic oils of menthol crystal, wintergreen, eucalyptus, camphor, and lavender. Keep away from eyes and mucous membranes, because it causes a burning sensation.

Liniment. Herbal liniments are made with alcohol and penetrating and warming herbs, which increase circulation to the area. You can make your own, or buy a commercial liniment at most drugstores and health food stores. Apply the liniment directly to the painful area and massage gently for 5 to 15 minutes, up to 4 times a day, preferably after a hot soak or bath. You should get relief from pain about twice as fast as without it. If you can't rub directly over the painful area, then rub around it with the liniment.

If you want to make your own liniment, make it before you actually need it, because it takes a week, and that's too long to wait when you're in pain.

Recipe: Liniment. Combine 4 tablespoons cayenne pepper, 3 tablespoons powdered myrrh, 3 tablespoons golden seal root powder, and 2 cups vodka in a bottle with a cork or tight-fitting lid. A brown or green bottle is preferable. Put a lid on the bottle, shake well, and keep it away from the sun. Shake the bottle once or twice a day for 7 to 14 days. On the last day, don't shake it; just pour out the liquid (not the sediment) into another bottle, and cork or close. Store away from the sun.

Note: Most herbalists begin their liniments and tinctures on or shortly after the new moon, and finish them before the full moon, because it is believed that the drawing power of the waxing moon helps to extract the active properties from the herbs.

Malachite. This is a dark green stone which often has a bull's-eye pattern. Malachite has the amazing ability to draw out pain—physical and emotional. The stone should be at least as large as the area that is painful.

Lie down and place the stone over the painful area and leave it there for at least 10 minutes. This could be done while doing crystal energization (See Index: Crystal energization).

Internal Treatments

Unflavored Gelatin. You can prevent a sore feeling in your muscles by taking 1 tablespoon of plain, unflavored powdered gelatin (available in any grocery store) and dissolving it in 1/2 cup of warm water. Drink this within an hour or two of the exertion. Presumably this remedy works by preventing the build-up of toxins in the muscles.

Bach Rescue Remedy. I carry this remedy with me wherever I go; it's useful in any crisis, large or small. It's good for physical pain and for emotional trauma. It's comforting for anything from a broken leg to final exams. One doctor gives his patients a few drops before surgery; he also gives it to his angina patients. This remedy enables the person who is hurt to calm down and deal with their problem, both physically and emotionally. When children are hurt, I give some to them, and then I give some to their parents. It's perfectly harmless, and can be combined with any medications.

Place 4 drops directly under the tongue, or in 1/4 cup of water or fruit juice. Repeat the dosage every 10 to 15 minutes as needed, and then gradually decrease the dosage. Often one dose is enough. If the person is unconscious, and if the remedy is in a base of alcohol (as it usually is), it can be put on the inside of the wrists, behind the earlobes, on the lips, or wherever the blood vessels are close to the surface, because the alcohol will be absorbed through the skin.

The Rescue Remedy and all the Bach Flower Remedies are more fully discussed in chapter 1.

Calcium. This is an effective pain-killer and it relieves muscle spasm, back pain, elbow pain, tendonitis, sprained shoulder, leg cramps, and dental pain. It is also useful for menstrual cramps and the pains of childbirth. And calcium is soothing to the nerves. When your blood calcium level goes down, your muscles tend to spasm. Normally, a woman's blood calcium level starts to drop 10 days before her menstrual period begins, which explains why so many women experience cramping.

Doses range from approximately 1000 to 2000 mg. of supplementary calcium per day. One to two tablets of 250 mg. can be taken every 2 or 3 hours while the pain is intense. After the pain eases, 1 to 3 tablets per day is usually enough. With chronic problems, you may need to maintain this dosage.

Valerian. This is an effective muscle relaxant and pain reliever. Valerian eases pain by depressing the central nervous system. Its name resembles the tranquilizer Valium (diazepam), but it is not related to it. Some people have a bad reaction to this herb, and complain of stomachache, nausea, dizziness, headaches, and bad dreams, so begin by using small quantities.

Valerian root can be taken alone, in powdered form, in 00 caps. Take 1 to 2 caps 1 to 3 times a day or as needed. This is the easiest way to take it, because it has a very strong odor and taste. However, some people prefer to use it in the granulated or shredded form, and to combine it with other herbs as a tea.

Recipe: Valerian, Scullcap, and Catnip Tea. Bring 2 cups water to a boil. Remove from the heat and add 1 teaspoon of each herb. Steep for 20 minutes. Reheat if desired, but do not boil.

Arnica. This is a homeopathic pain-reliever. It's so effective that I always carry some with me. Arnica can be taken in tablets of 6X potency. Children and pregnant women can use 30X potency. Use as instructed on the bottle.

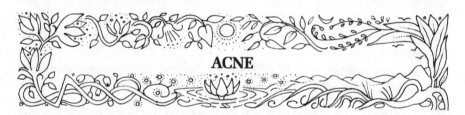

ACNE

This skin problem usually occurs during adolescence, though many adults also suffer from it. It is characterized by pimples and blackheads on the face, neck, and upper trunk.

During adolescence, there is increased hormonal activity as well as increased glandular secretions, including sebum from the sebaceous glands in the skin. Girls and women may have more trouble with acne during their periods.

In Chinese medicine, the skin is considered one of the organs of elimination, so when the colon is not functioning well, toxins may come out through the skin. The best results I've seen with acne have been from the use of blood cleansing teas (see chapter 4 on Eliminating Toxins) and acupuncture, which is used to regulate the endocrine glands. The following also have helped some individuals.

Cleansing. The formation of blackheads and whiteheads occurs when a hair follicle gets clogged by dirt or heavy cosmetics. Then the fatty material made by the gland at the root of the hair follicle accumulates, and a whitehead or blackhead forms under the skin. The dark color of blackheads is not dirt; it is caused by the discoloring effect of air on the fatty material. If this substance becomes infected, a pimple forms. Begin by washing the hands with soap and water; be sure to clean under the nails, because dirt will make the infection worse. Wash the affected skin. Then take a clean washcloth and hold it under very hot tap water. Apply this washcloth, as hot as possible, to each pimple. This will open the pores and soften the skin, making it easy to squeeze. After soaking for a minute or 2, the fatty material should come out easily. If not, leave them alone until they form a head, or else scarring or pitting may result. After this process is completed, apply cold water to the area. This will close the pores, which will help to prevent further infection. Apply witch hazel to each of the areas you worked on. This is a solution of the herb, witch hazel (*Hamamelis*), in water and alcohol. It is available in drugstores. Witch hazel causes the tissue to contract and the discharge to stop.

Diet. In some individuals, fatty foods seem to stimulate additional secretions and make the acne worse. Try to avoid chocolate, nuts, sharp cheese, ice cream, fatty meats, and fatty foods for a week. White sugar and white flour are also harmful to some individuals and should be avoided. If your condition improves during the week, you may have a sensitivity to these foods. Try re-introducing one food at a time, a few days apart, and observe your skin. You may find that some foods have a worse effect than others. You may have to repeat these experiments several times to be sure, because other factors can also affect your outbreaks. If your condition is particularly disturbing, consider a vegetarian diet, with a minimum of dairy products, nuts, and sugar, and plenty of fresh fruits, vegetables, and grains.

Vitamin B Complex. Emotional factors also affect some individuals. If your acne gets worse when you are under stress (final exams, arguments, financial worries), try treating the stress by taking supplementary vitamin B complex or brewer's yeast and vitamin C (see the section on Stress for more information). These vitamins will help you to cope better, and will help to relieve your stress. If your problems are serious, see a therapist.

When selecting a brand of vitamin B complex, be sure it has at least 10 mg. of B6 (pyridoxine). Many teenage women who have trouble with acne during their periods respond well to taking supplements of B6 for 1 week before and during their periods.

Niacin (Vitamin B3). This is another member of the B complex, but in this case, it should be taken separately because when it's included in B complex pills, it is usually in the form of niacinamide. For acne and headaches, niacin is specifically recommended, 100 mg., 3 times a day for 1 month. It will cause a hot flush within about 10 minutes, which goes away within about 15 minutes. This flush is part of the cure; it is caused by a dilation of blood vessels in the area and increased blood flow to the face.

Zinc. Taking at least 50 mg. per day of zinc gluconate has had dramatic results for many people.

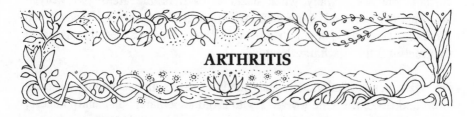

ARTHRITIS

This term covers more than 100 different types of joint diseases. The most common types are rheumatoid arthritis and osteoarthritis. Rheumatism is a general term for arthritis and is often applied to almost any pain in the joints or muscles. One or more joints may become swollen, painful, and inflamed. The symptoms may come and go, leaving no lasting disability. But if the disease progresses, there is degeneration of the joint, with permanent changes that produce deformities and immobility.

Arthritis and rheumatism are considered diseases of hardening, and according to Louise Hay in *Heal Your Body*, they reflect a sense of bitterness and resentment, and a feeling of being unloved. Arthritis in the fingers indicates that you are holding onto a desire to blame and punish.

Arthritis often responds well to acupuncture. In some cases, especially with arthritis of the fingers, just one treatment can last for 6 months or longer. It often helps to minimize or eliminate meat and dairy products from the diet.

There are many effective remedies for these disorders. I have not tried to distinguish which ones work best for specific kinds of arthritis.

Acids: Apple Cider Vinegar, Cherries, or Vitamin C. When the stomach doesn't produce enough hydrochloric acid, the body has difficulty breaking down calcium. Then the calcium doesn't get dissolved, and it piles up in the tissues and joints as calcium deposits, leading to arthritis. A hydrochloric acid deficiency may occur with digestive disorders or as a symptom of aging. Remedies that are high in natural acids are popular for these disorders.

An easy way to take apple cider vinegar is to bring 1 cup of water to a boil and add 1 to 2 tablespoons each of apple cider vinegar and honey (preferably raw). Drink 1 to 3 times per day.

Cherries can be eaten in any form: sweet, sour, fresh, canned, or frozen. People who consume lots of cherries report dramatic relief from arthritis.

For chronic arthritis, take 1000 mg. of vitamin C 4 times a day for relief from pain, an improved appetite and sense of well-being, and easier movement.

Alfalfa. This is one of the most amazing remedies for arthritis. Grind up alfalfa seeds (available in health food stores) and take 3 tablespoons of ground alfalfa seeds each day. It can be mixed with yogurt or whatever makes it palatable for you. Or take 7 or 8 tablets of alfalfa 2 or 3 times per day.

Comfrey Paste. You can make a poultice by applying comfrey paste directly over the swelling and then covering with gauze or cheesecloth. Leave it on for 24 hours, then apply a fresh poultice in the morning. Repeat until the swelling is gone.

To make comfrey paste, combine 1/4 cup honey and 1/4 cup olive oil in a blender and blend. Gradually add 1 cup chopped fresh comfrey leaves or 1/2 cup chopped fresh comfrey root and continue to blend until the mixture has a paste-like consistency. Then refrigerate as much as you need for the next 2 or 3 weeks. Freeze the remainder. Use as often as needed.

Comfrey Salve. You can use the salve just as you use the paste. Comfrey salve is available in most health food stores, but you can make your own by combining 1 cup vegetable oil and 1 cup fresh chopped comfrey leaves or 1/2 cup fresh chopped comfrey root in a saucepan. Simmer, covered, for about 30 minutes. Strain out the herbs, then slowly add 1/4 cup chopped beeswax and oil from 1 capsule vitamin E. Pour into container(s) and allow to cool and thicken.

Fresh Comfrey Poultice. Take fresh comfrey leaves and chop them or crush them with a mortar and pestle and apply directly to the painful area. Then cover with gauze or cheesecloth and leave it on all day. At night sprinkle with water—without removing the poultice—in order to moisten and bring out the active properties again. Leave it on all night. In the morning, apply a fresh poultice. Repeat until the swelling is gone.

Yucca. The Indians of the Southwest have long used the root of the yucca plant for arthritis. Many people with arthritis also have digestive and intestinal problems. Yucca contains saponin, which helps break down organic wastes. A daily dose of 2 to 8 tablets often gives relief to people with osteoarthritis and rheumatoid arthritis, and sometimes also improves the digestion.

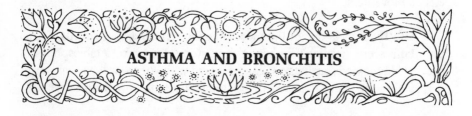

ASTHMA AND BRONCHITIS

The following remedies are effective for relieving the symptoms of asthma and bronchitis. When taken regularly, the lung tea and lung massage can strengthen the lungs and the immune system, and prevent further attacks from recurring—provided that your diet is good and you get plenty of fresh air and exercise.

Fresh air is necessary for the lungs to function properly, but warmth is also essential. In winter, keep a window open a crack and maintain the temperature at about 68°. At night, reduce the temperature to about 62° or less and use plenty of blankets (down comforters are nice). Walk outdoors in the fresh air at least once a day, but on cold days be sure to dress warmly.

Dry air (lack of humidity) is a prime offender in this condition. Wood or gas stoves and radiators should have a pot of water on them to keep the air from drying out. If you suffer from frequent congestion, a cold mist humidifier is a good investment. Vaporizers can also be used, but they give off hot, moist steam, whereas the humidifier gives off a cool mist, which is more effective. People who have asthma and bronchitis should try to avoid cigarette smoke.

According to Louise Hay, asthma occurs when people are oversensitive and feel stifled by a smothering kind of love. It can also be a sign of a suppressed need to cry. I find that asthma and bronchitis often occur when people are fearful and tend to hold their breath. This could be caused by living with highly unpredictable people, such as alcoholics.

Eucalyptus Oil. This powerful aromatic oil is very penetrating and effectively breaks through congestion, making it easier to breathe. It can be purchased in any drugstore. Add 1 teaspoon of eucalyptus oil to the water in a cold mist humidifier or vaporizer. (The instructions often caution not to add anything to the water, but I've been doing this for years and have had no problems. Just wash the humidifier and clean the filter after each use.)

If you don't have a humidifier or a vaporizer, you can bring 2 cups of water to a boil, remove the pot from the stove, and add 1/2 teaspoon of eucalyptus oil. Put your head over the pot, cover your head with a towel, and inhale the fumes. Continue for 5 to 10 minutes. You'll have to come up for air periodically.

If you have access to eucalyptus trees, use about 6 leaves and 6 seed pods in 2 cups of water. Simmer for 10 minutes, then inhale as described above. This water can be saved and used again several times.

Comfrey and Lobelia Tea. Comfrey increases your white blood cell count, which helps you to fight off infections. Lobelia relaxes the alveoli, the tiny air sacs within the lungs, so it can prevent or stop wheezing.

Recipe: Comfrey and Lobelia Tea. Bring 3 cups water to a boil and add 2 teaspoons comfrey leaves. Simmer for 10 minutes, then add 2 teaspoons each of lobelia and peppermint. Cover the pot and let it steep for 5 minutes. You can build up your resistance and strengthen your lungs by drinking 1 cup of this tea every other day.

Lobelia Inflata. This is a remedy that is made from lobelia by a homeopathic method. Lobelia relaxes the alveoli, the tiny air sacs within the lungs. It is very effective when taken at the first sign of wheezing. Use 6X potency, as instructed on the bottle. Lobelia Inflata can be obtained wherever homeopathic remedies are sold, or you can write to Standard Homeopathic Company (see Resources).

Ephedra Syrup. This is a powerful syrup that dilates the bronchioles— which is the same thing that more powerful medications do, but with fewer uncomfortable side effects. It is effective to use at the beginning of or during an attack.

Ephedra is a natural stimulant and can increase the heartbeat considerably. It should not be used by people who are taking standard medications. A child can be given ephedra, but you should monitor his or her heartbeat for about 30 minutes after giving the syrup. This can be done by holding the child calmly in your lap, with your hand over her or his heart, and counting the heartbeats for 30 seconds, then multiplying it by 2. Average pulsations in children over 7 are 80 to 90; at 1 to 7 years it is 80 to 120; infants have a heart rate 110 to 130 beats a minutes; and at birth, it is 130 to 160.

In the recipe that follows, catnip is combined with ephedra to provide a calming counter effect. If the pulse exceeds the average by more than 10 beats, then further sedation is needed. Please see the section on Nervous Tension.

Recipe: Ephedra Syrup. Bring 2 cups of water to a boil. Add 3 heaping tablespoons granulated ephedra or 1 medium-size handful ephedra twigs. Simmer for 10 minutes and remove from the heat. Add 2 tablespoons catnip. Brew in a covered pot for 5 more minutes.

Dose: Give babies 3 to 4 drops in an eyedropper; give small children 1 to 2 teaspoons; adults take 3 to 4 teaspoons. Wait at least 30 minutes before taking more. This is a very potent syrup.

Note: There are various *Ephedra* species. It's also known as desert tea, Mormon tea, and ma huang. The latter is *Ephedra sinensis* or Chinese ephedra, and it is more potent than American ephedra. So if you use ma huang, use about three-quarters as much (if the recipe calls for 1 teaspoon, use 3/4 teaspoon; if it calls for 1 tablespoon, use 2 teaspoons).

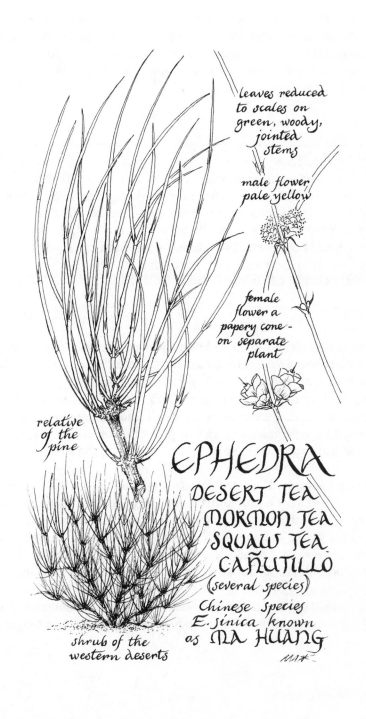

leaves reduced
to scales on
green, woody,
jointed
stems

male flower
pale yellow

female
flower a
papery cone -
on separate
plant

relative
of the
pine

EPHEDRA
DESERT TEA
MORMON TEA
SQUAW TEA
CAÑUTILLO
(several species)
Chinese species
E. sinica known
as MA HUANG

shrub of the
western deserts

Lung Tea. This tea is good for any form of lung congestion. Taken regularly, at least 1 cup every other day, it will help to strengthen your lungs and build up your immune system. Taken during an attack of asthma or bronchitis, it will help to raise the phlegm, clear the lungs, and strengthen your resistance.

Recipe: Lung Tea. Bring 6 cups water to a boil. Add 1 tablespoon mullein and 1 tablespoon coltsfoot. Simmer for 10 minutes, then add 1 tablespoon cornsilk (from Indian corn), 1 tablespoon lobelia, and 2 tablespoons peppermint. Brew for 5 minutes, then strain. Add as much honey as you want. When you have a cold, drink as much as possible. People who have chronic congestion can strengthen their lungs by drinking 1 or 2 cups every day.

No Wheeze Tea. Master herbalist and author Jeanne Rose has prepared a very effective tea for asthma called No Wheeze Tea. It contains black tea, elecampane root, fritillary, comfrey leaf, eucalyptus leaf, yerba santa leaf, ginseng root, orange peel, orange oil, and mullein flower. The amount of comfrey leaf in this tea is so small that I doubt it would be harmful to anyone—though pregnant women may prefer to avoid it. The tea is available from the San Francisco Herb and Natural Food Company.

Lung Massage. If you feel an attack coming on—or just to strengthen the lungs—it is very useful to firmly massage the arm along the acupuncture meridian of the lung, starting from the shoulder and going down to the inside edge of the thumbnail. To strengthen the lungs, use this massage 3 times a week for 2 weeks, then twice a week for 2 weeks, then once a week for 2 weeks, then one more time 2 weeks later. See illustration.

Citrine. This beautiful yellow stone is useful for asthma. At the first sign of wheezing, place a small tumbled citrine under your tongue.

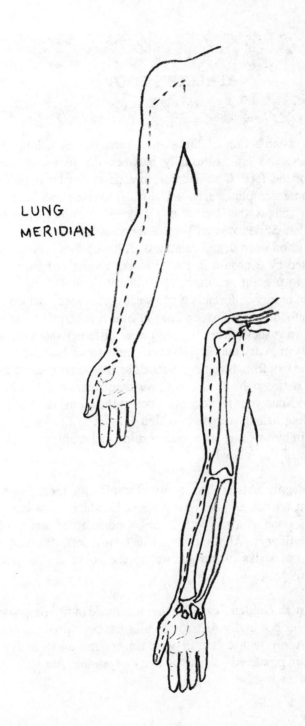

LUNG
MERIDIAN

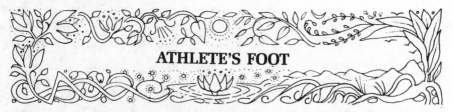

ATHLETE'S FOOT

This is a fungus infection of the skin, which causes itching, redness, scaling, blisters, and cracks, usually between the toes and sometimes on the soles of the feet. It sometimes spreads to the heels and toenails and may become complicated by additional moisture and bacteria. The most common fungus that causes this is yeast (*candida albicans*), the same fungus that causes vaginal yeast infections.

Fungi thrive on warmth and dampness. Athlete's foot is contagious and easily contracted by exposure in public locker rooms and showers. Wear rubber thongs to prevent getting or spreading it.

You will be more comfortable if you wear cotton socks, which breathe, rather than synthetic socks, which hold in moisture. Don't wear socks at night. Change your socks every day, and wear different shoes on alternate days to allow them to dry out. Try to avoid tennis shoes because the rubber soles prevent the foot from breathing. Sandals are helpful because they enable air to circulate between the toes. In cold weather, wear sandals with 2 pairs of cotton socks. Keep your feet dry and open to the air as much as possible.

Athlete's foot usually responds within 1 week to the following home remedies. Begin by washing your feet morning and night, dry thoroughly, then apply one of the following.

White Vinegar. This is the remedy of choice for most fungal infections because it creates an acid environment in which yeast can't thrive. Combine 1 teaspoon vinegar with 2 tablespoons water and apply with cotton or your fingers. Allow to dry; don't rinse off. It's also a good idea to rinse your socks in vinegar water; use about 2 tablespoons per gallon of water.

Liniment with Golden Seal. The liniment made of myrrh, golden seal, and cayenne described under Aches and Pains has been used effectively for athlete's foot. Apply with cotton or your fingers and allow to dry. Alternatively, use plain powdered golden seal as a *foot powder.* Just sprinkle about 1/4 teaspoon in each shoe.

Aloe Vera. Apply the gel from the leaves of the fresh plant and allow to dry.

Comfrey Paste. This mixture combines the healing properties of vitamin E, honey, and allantoin, the active ingredient in comfrey, which causes rapid healing of cells. All of these substances have been used effectively for athlete's foot. To make comfrey paste, combine 1/4 cup honey and 1/4 cup olive oil in a blender and blend. Gradually add 1 cup chopped fresh comfrey leaves or 1/2 cup chopped fresh comfrey root and continue to blend until the mixture has a paste-like consistency. Then refrigerate as much as you need for the next 2 or 3 weeks and freeze the rest.

Urine. Urine is astringent and acidic. When the body is attacked, it manufactures antibodies to fight off the foreign invader. These antibodies can be found in the urine. By using the urine externally, we're helping the body to carry on a battle that it must otherwise do internally.

This method is extremely effective, not only for simple athlete's foot, but also for cracked heels and fungus under the toenails (the latter, however may return in 2 or 3 weeks and require a second treatment). Most people apply this remedy by urinating on their feet while in the shower. Some prefer to urinate into a small jar, mix it half and half with wine or vinegar and apply with a cotton swab. The feet can may be rinsed with plain water after this treatment.

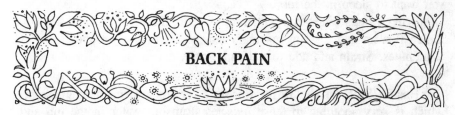

BACK PAIN

Your mattress is vitally important; make sure you are sleeping on a firm one. If you have a water bed, you should probably get rid of it; most chiropractors say they are harmful for the back. Electric blankets are also discouraged because they interfere with the body's natural alignment. If you have a sagging box spring, cut a board the size of your mattress (3/8-inch plywood works well) and put it between the mattress and the box spring. Or remove the box spring entirely and put the mattress directly on the floor. Or get a new mattress.

Chiropractors are back specialists, and they can usually work wonders with back problems. If the following remedies are not adequate, see a good chiropractor. Back problems can lead to numerous other ailments, including fatigue, irritability, and sciatica.

In the language of the body, back pain suggests that you have been carrying a heavy load, taking on too many responsibilities. Before trying the remedies listed below, consider lightening your load; don't allow yourself to be a beast of burden.

Yoga. Some of the asanas (exercises) that are useful are the cobra, backward bend, locust, bow, plough, full twist, elbow-to-knee, and alternate leg pull. These asanas can be found in most books on yoga. They are described in detail, with good photographs, in Richard Hittleman's *Yoga 29 Day Exercise Plan* (Bantam Books).

Thermophore. The thermophore is excellent for back problems. Unfortunately, the price of this wonderful device is a bit high, but anyone with a chronic back problem can hardly afford to be without one. For a more complete description, see Index.

Herbal Bath. This sweet-smelling bath is a wonderful way to alleviate back pain. Usually 25 minutes is long enough to stay in this bath, unless you want to sleep in the tub.

Bring 4 cups water to a boil, remove from the heat, and add 2/3 cup linden flowers and 1/3 cup rosemary leaves. Cover the pot and steep for 10 minutes. Strain and add to the bath water.

Epsom Salts in the Bath. Epsom salts are a form of magnesium, which is very soothing to tense muscles. Run hot water in the tub and add about 1 cup of salts. When they dissolve, adjust the temperature and run a normal bath, soaking as long as you like.

Color. The color blue is calming, soothing, and anti-inflammatory, so it is particularly good for soothing an aching back. Since red is stimulating and irritating, it should be avoided. One chiropractor routinely advises his patients with back pain to avoid wearing red shirts. I've found that light blue shirts work well for back pain.

Pain in the upper back, between the shoulder blades, relates to the heart and is often caused by problems of love. If that is the case, pink or green may be soothing to wear. Pain at the small of the back involves your sense of power, and the feeling of having some kind of monkey on your back. Pain in the lower back relates to your foundations. Such pain may occur when you feel you are losing your support system.

If you have access to a colored lamp, try lying under one of these colors for 5 to 30 minutes, once or twice a day to relieve nerve and muscle tension and inflammation. It's also good to bring these colors into your environment in the form of flowers, wall hangings, or in any way that appeals to you.

Vitamin C. Massive doses of vitamin C have been used effectively for back pain, including such serious problems as scoliosis (unnatural curvature of the spine), fractured vertebrae, displaced vertebrae, and disintegrating discs. Vitamin C plays an essential role in the formation of collagen, the cement-like substance that holds together the cells of bones, cartilage, and muscles. When the collagen is weak, the bones and muscles lose their elasticity and rupture easily, which can lead to anything from a stiff back to a disintegrating disc.

Depending on the seriousness of your problem, and your individual reaction to vitamin C, dosages can range from 500 to 2000 mg., 2 to 4 times a day. (See chapter 5 for more information on Vitamin C.)

Valerian. This is an effective muscle relaxant and pain reliever. Valerian eases pain by depressing the central nervous system. Some people have a bad reaction to this herb, and complain of stomachache, nausea, dizziness, headaches, and bad dreams, so begin by using small quantities.

Valerian root can be taken alone, in powdered form, in 00 caps. Take 1 to 2 caps 1 to 3 times a day or as needed. This is the easiest way to take it, because it has a very strong odor and taste. However, some people prefer to use it in the granulated or shredded form, and to combine it with other herbs as a tea.

Recipe: Valerian, Scullcap, and Catnip Tea. Bring 2 cups water to a boil. Remove from the heat and add 1 teaspoon of each herb. Steep for 20 minutes. Reheat if desired, but do not boil.

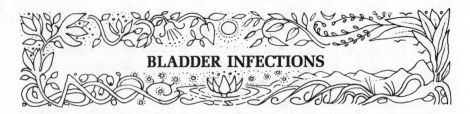

BLADDER INFECTIONS

If you have trouble urinating, you may have a bladder infection, but it's hard to be sure because the symptoms—burning urine, frequent urination, and pain in the bladder—can be an indication of many things, including venereal or kidney disease. Be sure to get a diagnosis from a doctor.

Since urine is a good medium for bacterial growth, and since the urethra is close to the vagina, women can become infected during intercourse, so women are more susceptible to bladder infections than men. If you are prone to having bladder infections, be sure to urinate before intercourse, and then urinate again after intercourse, to wash out the bacteria. Dilute your urine by drinking at least 8 glasses of liquid per day. After a bowel movement, wipe from front to back, to avoid contaminating your urethra.

When you are run down, you are more susceptible to getting an infection, so get plenty of rest and cut down on strenuous work. Avoid drinks with caffeine, such as coffee, black tea, cocoa, and soft drinks. Also avoid alcohol.

Bladder infections are most likely to occur when you are feeling angry about something, or when you are holding back, afraid to let go.

Cranberry Juice. Drink at least 1/2 cup of cranberry juice 4 times a day. Cranberry juice is especially effective for cleaning out the kidneys and bladder. If you don't like cranberry, try 1 cup of cranapple juice 4 times a day.

Vitamin C. Take 1000 mg. of vitamin C 3 times a day to make your urine acidic so that bacteria will not grow in it. See chapter 5 for more information on Vitamin C.

Golden Seal. On the first day only, take 2 gelatin capsules (size 00) of powdered golden seal root followed by a half glass of warm water.

Bladder Tea. This tea is effective in treating bladder infections. If this tea causes an upset stomach (especially in children or pregnant women), eliminate the echinacea and/or yarrow. Drink 1 cup a day for a week.

> **Recipe: Bladder Tea.** Bring 3 cups of water to a boil and add 1 tablespoon echinacea root. Simmer for 20 minutes, then remove from the heat and add 2 teaspoons yarrow flowers, 2 teaspoons bearberry (uva-ursi), 2 teaspoons cornsilk (from Indian corn), and 1 teaspoon juniper berries. Steep for 15 minutes in a covered container, then strain. Store the unused portion in the refrigerator.
>
> If you cannot obtain or cannot use 1 or 2 of these herbs, increase the other herbs, and the tea should still be effective.

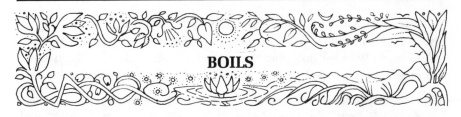

BOILS

Boils are red, swollen, painful areas on the skin that resemble overgrown pimples. They occur mostly on the neck and buttocks.

Avoid scratching boils, since this can cause the release of pus, which then spreads to healthy areas of the skin and may cause new boils to erupt. The bacterium that causes boils is staph, and once it gets into the body, it can be very hard to get rid of, causing recurrent boils and possibly infecting others. This is why an internal treatment is often needed as well as an external one.

Boils can be painful because the swelling causes pressure on the nerve endings. This can be particularly disconcerting if the boils are on your bottom. Boils are often a sign that resistance is low, which may be the result of illness or of poor nutrition.

Boils tend to occur when a person is boiling mad about something. The location of the boil should give further information. For example, a boil on the buttocks could mean that you are experiencing someone or something as a royal pain in the butt.

External Treatments

When treating a boil externally, apply moist heat as often as possible. This increases the blood flow to the area and helps bring the boil to a head, so it will drain by itself. It also keeps the surface soft and free of scabs that can close the skin and trap the infection. The soaking can be done with a clean washcloth dipped in hot water, as hot as possible, and applied repeatedly for 10 to 15 minutes, 3 to 6 times a day. Whenever the washcloth cools, dip it in hot water again. Alternatively, the following home remedies may be used to further the drawing process.

Hot Black Tea Bag. Black tea contains tannic acid, which has strong drawing powers. The tea bag helps hold the heat.

Plantain Poultice. When fresh, this herb has great drawing powers. The plant is a weed that grows on most unsprayed lawns and meadows. (See Index: Insect Bites for information on plantain). Macerate a leaf of plantain and tape it over the boil, after soaking. Replace several times a day.

Burdock Soak. Make a strong tea by boiling 2 cups of water and adding 4 tablespoons burdock root. Simmer for 20 minutes. Strain. Then dip the washcloth into this decoction instead of hot water. Be sure to keep the decoction tolerably hot.

Internal Treatments

The internal remedies are for cleansing the blood and ridding the body of staph. They are most important to use if you have had more than 1 boil in the last few months.

Oil Of Bitter Orange. This remedy is used by naturopaths for staph, and I've seen it clear up boils that would not respond even to antibiotics. Bitter oranges grow in Africa, and they are too strong to eat. The oil is very powerful. Take 4 drops in about 1/2 cup of orange juice, 3 times a day (3 drops for children). Use until all symptoms are gone, and then for another 2 to 3 days. Most cases clear up with one 1/4-ounce bottle, in 3 to 7 days, but if it's a long-standing case, you may need up to 3 bottles. This remedy is available in some herb and health food stores, or you can order it from Nature's Herbs (see Resources).

Echinacea and Burdock Tea. Burdock has a bitter flavor. Drink 1 cup, 3 times a day until symptoms are gone, and then 1 cup per day for another 3 days.

Recipe: Echinacea and Burdock Tea. Bring 4 cups of water to a boil and add 2 teaspoons echinacea root and 2 teaspoons burdock root. Cover and simmer for 20 minutes.

Sassafras Tea. Sassafras has a rather pleasant flavor. *Note*: Some people hesitate to drink sassafras tea, because of an article that appeared in the *Journal of the American Medical Association*, which stated that sassafras tea can cause cancer. Another article was written in rebuttal by Norman Farnsworth et. al., from the Department of Pharmacology and Pharmacognosy at the University of Illinois. This second article was submitted to *JAMA* but was not published by them. The article stated that while sassafras *oil* could, in fact, cause cancer, the oil is not water-soluble. Therefore, sassafras tea does not contain more than a minute amount of the oil and will not cause cancer unless you fail to strain your tea and then chew on the pieces of bark.

Recipe: Sassafras Tea. Bring 3 1/2 cups of water to a boil and add 1 tablespoon sassafras. Cover and simmer for 20 minutes. Drink 1 to 3 cups a day. It is a blood cleanser.

When to Call a Medical Worker

If the patient is an infant or young child or an elderly person; if the boil is on or above the upper lip, on the nose, on the scalp, or in the outer ear (these areas have easy access to the brain); if the boil is in the armpit or groin (these areas have easy access to the bloodstream and can cause blood-poisoning); if the boil is in the breast of a nursing woman; or if there is a fever of over 100° F., consult a medical worker.

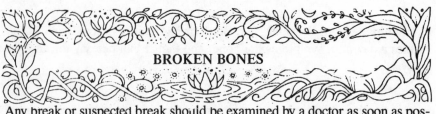

BROKEN BONES

Any break or suspected break should be examined by a doctor as soon as possible. The following remedies are meant to be used in conjunction with the usual procedures for broken bones, to relieve the pain and to speed healing. A broken nose, toe, rib, and various other chipped bones cannot be put in a cast or treated by conventional methods, but they will respond beautifully to the following remedies. Pain is eased, and breaks heal far more rapidly than anticipated.

When casts are used, I find it's best that they be removed at the earliest possible time to facilitate gentle massage, baths, whirlpools, and mild exercise to the joints. These procedures have been used successfully by the Chinese, as described in *Away With All Pests* by Dr. Felix Manne. The early mobilization of broken limbs enables them to heal faster, and with virtually no resulting handicaps. But one must be very conscientious to avoid weight-bearing on a leg that is not yet fully mended and to avoid using an arm that is not yet truly knit.

Your bones are the foundation of your body and your existence. A broken bone may indicate that you are feeling insecure and unstable. Louise Hay associates this with rebelling against authority.

Comfrey is a wonder-herb when it comes to healing broken bones. Its folk-name is knitbone, which is well deserved. Taken internally, it hastens healing by causing an increase in white blood cells, which strengthens the body's self-defense system. It's also high in calcium, which is important for the healing of bone tissue. Comfrey reduces swelling, enabling the bones to join together and knit properly. Comfrey contains allantoin, which accelerates cell proliferation, stimulates tissue formation, and hastens wound healing. Leeches secrete allantoin, which is why they used to put them on wounds, to promote rapid healing. For external use, I use comfrey root, because it is higher in allantoin.

So there are plenty of reasons why comfrey is good for you. But studies have shown that comfrey contains cancer-causing substances. (See the introduction to this chapter.) For this reason, I use only the leaves for tea, and I limit the daily use of comfrey to a 2-week maximum. I think it would be foolish to avoid comfrey altogether, because it is one of our finest medicinal herbs.

External Treatments

Comfrey. A good comfrey paste or salve should be applied liberally over the area of the break, and then covered with a suitable bandage, since comfrey does stain. It will help relieve the pain and will significantly speed up healing. Even if there is a cast, as long as the cast is permeable and not too far from the skin, the paste or salve can be put on the cast and it will absorb into the skin and then down to the bone. A fresh dressing should be applied once or twice a day. It can be left on for a minimum of 15 minutes and preferably for 1 hour, and then removed if necessary. Ideally, leave it on for 24 hours. A fresh dressing should be applied each day.

Recipe: Comfrey Paste. Combine 1/4 cup honey (preferably raw) and 1/4 cup olive oil in a blender. Blend for 1 minute, then remove the center piece from the blender lid, and gradually add 1 cup chopped fresh comfrey leaves, or 1/2 cup fresh chopped comfrey root, or 1/4 cup powdered comfrey root. Blend and add comfrey until the mixture has a paste-like consistency. Then refrigerate as much as you may need for the next 2 or 3 weeks. Freeze extra to use during the winter. Use as often as needed.

Recipe: Comfrey Salve. Combine 1 cup vegetable oil and 1 cup fresh chopped comfrey leaves or 1/2 cup fresh chopped comfrey root in a saucepan over low heat. Simmer, covered, for 1/2 hour. Strain out the herb, then slowly add 1/4 cup chopped beeswax and oil from 1 capsule vitamin E. Place in container(s) and allow to cool and thicken.

Green Jade. Jade helps broken bones to heal faster. Whenever possible, tape a piece of jade over the broken bone. When there is a cast, tuck a thin piece or two of jade under the cast. Jade is warm, soothing, and protective.

Moisturizer. When a limb is immobilized for over a week, the skin begins to dry out. Hospitals use moisturizers to keep the flesh healthy and to prevent dryness and itching. But these moisturizers usually contain mineral oil, which is absorbed into the blood where it attaches to oil-soluble vitamins, including vitamin A, which is essential for healthy skin. It carries these vitamins out in the urine. I have found that lotions that are high in aloe vera are very effective as moisturizers.

Internal Treatments

As explained above, comfrey tea will increase your white blood cells and strengthen your body's self-defense system. Drink 1 cup a day on alternate days for up to 2 weeks. Pregnant women and children under 6 years old should avoid this tea.

Recipe: Comfrey Tea. Bring 6 cups water to a boil, then add 2 tablespoons comfrey leaves. Simmer for 10 minutes. If desired, add 2 tablespoons peppermint. Steep for 5 minutes. Refrigerate.

Calcium and Magnesium. Both of these minerals are vital in the formation of bones. Take at least 1000 mg. calcium and 500 mg. magnesium a day.

Vitamin C. Take at least 1000 mg. vitamin C a day to aid in bone formation.

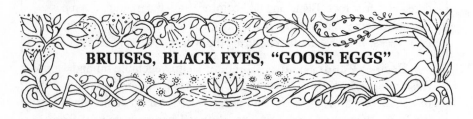

BRUISES, BLACK EYES, "GOOSE EGGS"

People who tend to get banged up are often suffering from a desire to harm themselves. They usually have a deep sense of guilt.

Ice Pack. Wrap a few ice cubes in a towel, and apply *immediately* to the injured area. Ideally, wrap the ice cubes in a rag and hammer them into chips, then put the chips in a towel. Chips or small cubes will mold to the injured area more easily than large cubes.

Rub It. This may sound strange, but rubbing a part of the body that has been banged up (this does not apply to the eyes) helps to relieve pain and prevent swelling—as long as the skin is not broken or scraped. Rubbing works by increasing circulation to the area. Keep your fingers in one place and rub in a circular motion. Don't rub back and forth over the skin, but stimulate the tissue beneath the skin.

Castor Oil. Castor oil increases the circulation to the area where it is applied and prevents or takes away pain, swelling, and even the discoloration of bruises and black eyes. It is made from the oil of the castor bean, and it is available at any drugstore. Just dab it on. For best results, apply about 3 times a day, until the healing is complete. If some oil accidentally gets into the eye, don't worry, because it is not harmful to the eyes. Keep it away from children, because it's a powerful purgative when taken internally.

Green Poultices. The macerated leaves of plantain, comfrey, or cabbage can be applied to the painful area. Plantain is a common weed, found on most unsprayed lawns. Comfrey is a popular herb, and many people grow it in their gardens. If you are healthy, the simplest way to macerate the leaves is to chew them (saliva also has healing properties). Or they can be chopped fine and mashed with a mortar and pestle, or a clean rock in a bowl. Clean the area and then apply the macerated leaves to the bump or bruise, and cover with gauze, using adhesive tape to keep it in place. This is a good remedy to use even when the skin is scraped or cut.

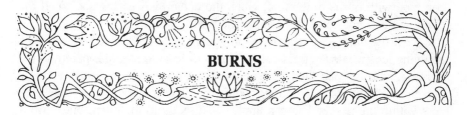

BURNS

Burns tend to occur when we feel like we have been burned by someone. They are also a way that our bodies have of telling us to slow down.

Since medical workers commonly refer to the degree of a burn, it is useful to understand this terminology. First degree burns are minor burns that do not cause blistering. The skin is reddened, and only the first layer of skin (the epidermis) is damaged.

Second degree burns are fairly serious burns that cause blisters and damage 2 layers of skin (the epidermis and the dermis). Do not break the blisters, because they are a kind of natural dressing. If they do break by themselves, allow the overlying skin to remain as a wet dressing. If the blisters are in an area of the body that is dirty, wash with soap and water and if it's likely to get dirty again, apply sterile gauze and keep it clean. If signs of infection appear (pus, bad smell, fever, swollen lymph glands), apply compresses of warm salt water and take give plenty of vitamin C. It may be desirable to get some neosporin, which is an over-the-counter antibiotic ointment. You may want to see a doctor.

Third degree burns are usually deep burns that destroy the skin and expose raw or charred flesh, which may be white or black. It usually involves the deep layer of the skin (the subcutaneous). Third degree burns also refer to any burn that covers a large portion of the body (an area that is larger than 2 of the person's own hands). Don't treat third degree burns yourself unless you have all the necessary home remedies, and you feel confident (and the person who is burned feels confident in you), or if you cannot reach a medical worker. The responsibility is yours. If you don't feel confident, it is better to get the burn into cold water and then wrap it with a very clean cloth and get the help of a medical worker.

The following combines first aid advice with the most popular and effective home remedies.

If you have been burned with boiling liquid, immediately pull off all wet clothes, or else the skin will continue to cook inside the cloth (this is common with burns to the feet, when the person is wearing socks). If the clothing does not come off easily, cut it off carefully.

Cool the burn immediately by plunging it into cold or ice water, or by applying ice (whatever feels best). This will help to stop the pain and the burning, and it is one thing that all authorities agree upon. It can actually prevent the burn from becoming worse, because it stops the burning process within the tissue. You can apply ice directly to the burn, but move it around gently rather than keeping it in one place because the ice can harm the skin tissue. Continue to cool the burn for up to 1 hour or more.

Stay calm. Although burns are serious, if they are treated properly, they should heal well. Give tender loving care. Fear is potentially more harmful than the burn itself. Relate to the person with your whole being. Encourage them to breathe deeply, and do so yourself. Explain that deep breathing helps bring blood and oxygen to the brain and the heart, which will help combat fear and prevent shock.

A person with a third degree burn should be given the following solution: 1 quart of water, 1/2 teaspoon salt, 1/2 teaspoon baking soda, 2 to 3 tablespoons sugar or honey, and 2 to 3 tablespoons orange or lemon juice, if available. This will help to replace body fluids that are lost through the oozing burn. The burned person should drink this as often as possible, especially until he or she is urinating frequently.

For Fear and Pain

Arnica. This is an effective homeopathic pain-reliever. It can be taken internally, in pills of 6x potency. These pills can be found in some herb and health food stores or ordered from the Standard Homeopathic Company (see Resources). Use as directed on the bottle.

Bach Rescue Remedy. This is always excellent for situations of fear or pain. The burned person and the attendants should take 4 drops under the tongue every 5 minutes. As the pain and fear lessen, reduce the dosage to 10 minutes, 15 minutes, or as needed. If the person is unconscious, the drops can be placed at the insides of their wrists, or behind the earlobes, where it will be absorbed into the blood. For more information on the Bach Rescue Remedy, see chapter 1. It is important for the attendant(s) to take the remedy, too, because if you are calm, you will impart your confidence to the person who is burned.

Tylenol or Aspirin. Either one of these can be used to relieve pain if arnica and Rescue Remedy are not available.

Shock

With a serious burn, one of the worst dangers is shock. There are 2 main causes of shock: 1) There may be so much blood loss in the injured area that it causes a leak in the circulatory system, and the blood pressure drops so that there's not enough pressure to carry the blood to the brain and other organs; or 2) if there is great fear, the body may be so stunned that it loses control of the circulatory system: the blood vessels relax and expand (dilate) instead of pushing the blood through. Then the blood pressure drops and the vital organs are deprived of their blood supply. In either situation, a lack of blood to the brain can cause brain damage within 7 minutes. A lack of blood to the heart can eventually cause death. So the alleviation of fear and the replacement of fluids is a vital part of treating any serious burn. The symptoms of shock are cold and clammy skin; fast, weak pulse that increases in rate; falling blood pressure; paleness in face; dizziness; nausea; dilated pupils; restlessness and anxiety; progressively slurred speech; and loss of memory.

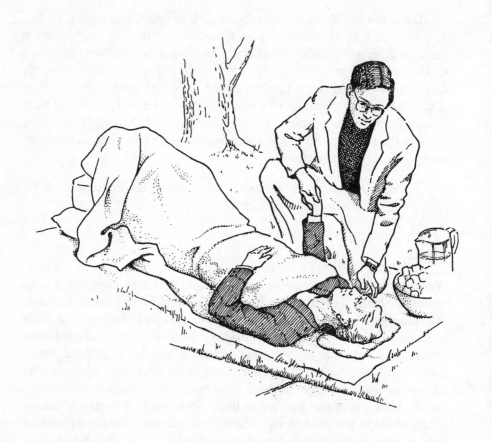

In addition to staying calm and giving remedies for fear and pain described above, the following first aid measures are advisable.

The person should lie down, with his or her legs elevated 12 inches or more (unless there is an injury to the head or chest). This helps bring the blood to the brain and heart. Use sheets or blankets to keep the person comfortably warm, but not hot. Small amounts of water or fluid (as described above) should be given unless there is a possibility of abdominal injury or vomiting, or if the person is unconscious. Sucking on an ice cube can be comforting, especially with a burn. The pulse should be taken every 5 minutes.

For Healing Serious Burns

Cleaning the Burn. Wash your hands. After you remove the burned area from the cold water, examine it to see if it is dirty. If it is, it will have to be washed with soap and water. This should be done gently, but it will probably be painful. (If you are afraid of causing pain by treating the burn properly, then you should take the injured person to a medical worker.) After you wash the burn, pat it dry with a clean towel.

Dressing the Burn. Most first aid books caution against applying any kind of salve, oil, butter, grease, or lubricant to the burn, but I've worked in clinics with many medical workers, and we've found the following remedies to be extremely effective, even with third degree burns. We apply one of the following to sterile gauze or cloth, and then wrap the burned area. This method is preferable to applying anything directly to the burned area, because it minimizes touching the area, which is generally painful. Cleanliness is one of the most important things in treating a serious wound. If you don't have sterile gauze, use strips of clean linen or a clean diaper. A clean cloth can be reasonably sterilized by ironing before use.

The dressing should be changed every day. When the burn no longer hurts and has begun to heal, it can be left exposed to the air, without dressing. Any of the following can be used. Some people like to alternate between them, believing that each contributes in its own way to the healing process.

External Treatments

Aloe Vera. A succulent plant that grows in the heat of the desert, aloe attracts moisture to itself even under inhospitable conditions. It's not surprising that the aloe would be an excellent moisturizer and coolant, giving quick relief to the scorched.

Aloe is an attractive houseplant and needs little attention. It grows in indirect sunlight and needs watering only every 7 to 10 days. To use medicinally, cut off the tip of one of the lower leaves. The plant will quickly seal over and heal its own wound. Peel back the skin of the leaf, and apply the thick jelly directly to the burn. The plant may be purchased from some florists. The bottled gel is also available in health food stores, but it is not as effective.

Vitamin E (preferably alpha tocopherols). Vitamin E is popular for burns, and often helps to prevent scarring. In addition to taking it internally (see below), it is applied directly to the burned area after the burn has cooled (if applied while the burn is still hot, the oil may cook on the skin, making it even more painful). Puncture a capsule of vitamin E oil with a pin at both ends, and squeeze the oil directly onto the burn. Some people use vitamin E ointment, which is available in health food stores.

Vitamin E is well known for its remarkable ability to prevent or eliminate scarring. Blood carries oxygen to all the tissues of the body. When a deep burn occurs, the tiny blood capillaries are injured, and oxygen can't get to the cells. Scar tissue is the kind of tissue that forms in the absence of sufficient oxygen. Vitamin E is helpful because it is a biological antioxidant: It prevents oxygen from being used up quickly in the bloodstream by slowing down the oxidation of lipids (fats) in the bloodstream. While burns are healing, the surfaces are likely to be red and angry looking and raised above the surface of the skin. As the skin grows in and the area heals, this will subside. Even infected burns can be treated the same way and will respond within 4 to 5 days.

But there is a wide range of response to vitamin E. For some, it is a miracle drug. For others, it is useful, but not as good as other remedies.

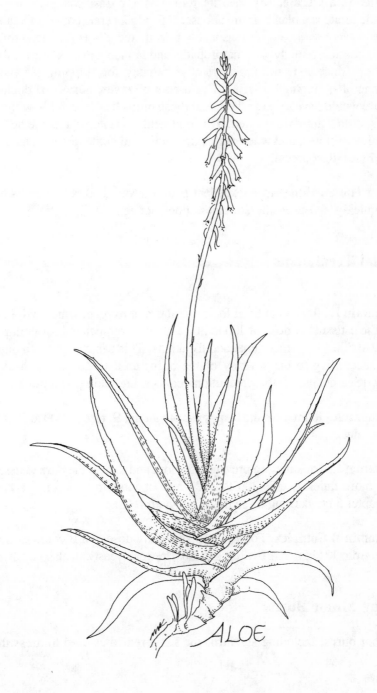

ALOE

Calendula Cerate. My favorite remedy for burns, calendula is pot marigold; cerate is a bland ointment base. Calendula cerate comes in a tube, it's easy to carry with you, it's reasonably priced, and it lasts for a long time. This is a popular remedy with naturopaths and homeopaths. I always carry it with me since it is the most effective remedy for stopping pain and preventing blistering and scarring. I've used it on severe burns that doctors were sure would have to be grafted, and those burns healed quickly without scar tissue. Just apply as needed. This ointment is available at some health food and herb stores, and wherever naturopathic and homeopathic remedies are sold (see Resources).

Raw Honey. Honey is an excellent pain reliever. The skin absorbs the honey quickly and even the stickiness does not remain.

Internal Treatments

Vitamin E . Take vitamin E for optimal use of oxygen, which will help prevent scar tissue. A dose of 100 to 300 I.U. is recommended for children and 200 to 800 I.U. is recommended for adults. This can be used as a daily dosage, according to the severity of the burn, until the burn has healed entirely. (See chapter 5 for precautions concerning taking Vitamin E.)

Vitamin A. To improve the body's use of vitamin E, take 25,000 to 50,000 I. U. per day.

Vitamin C. For stress, to prevent infection, and to help the burned tissue to heal more quickly, take 100 to 1000 mg. of vitamin C 4 times a day. (See chapter 5 concerning large doses of vitamin C.)

Vitamin B Complex. For stress, take a daily dose of a B complex that contains from 10 to 50 mg. B1, B2, and B6. Brewer's yeast can also be taken.

Healing Minor Burns

For minor burns, including sunburn, the same remedies used to dress the serious burn can be applied directly to the skin. It's not necessary to cover with gauze or cloth, though some people find that it helps relieve the pain, and it keeps the wound clean.

Burns Around Joints

If a person has been burned between the fingers, or in the armpit, or at other joints, use gauze pads covered with one of the remedies listed under External Treatments (above), between the burned surfaces, to prevent the skin around the joints from growing together as it heals. Also, fingers, arms, legs, and toes should be straightened completely several times a day while healing. This is painful, but it helps to prevent stiff scars which later make it impossible to properly bend and straighten the joints.

When to See a Medical Worker

If you are afraid, and don't feel competent to treat the burn yourself, particularly if it involves the face or hands or feet, if it is a third degree burn, if there is infection, or if it continues to be painful for more than 48 hours, see a medical worker. If there are signs of shock which don't improve or get worse, see a medical worker immediately.

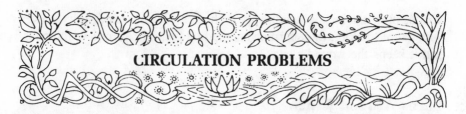

CIRCULATION PROBLEMS

Coldness in the extremities may be a slight annoyance, or it may be a serious problem. The sensation of cold may change to that of numbness, tingling, pins and needles, or even burning and pain. This is most common in the feet, but it also occurs in the hands.

The most common way to deal with this problem is to wear long johns, cotton or wool socks, woolen mittens, and a hat (a lot of body heat is lost through the head). Avoid socks made of synthetics and don't wear them at night; try a heating pad instead. Red long johns, socks, etc., will heat you up faster than blue ones—especially if you can see them. Orange and yellow are also warming colors.

Many people have found that sandals with ski socks or cotton socks actually keep their feet warmer than boots, although keeping dry can be a problem. Sandals are sometimes warmer because boots cut off circulation to the toes.

A warm bath followed by a cool one will increase circulation. Cold hands or feet heat up quickly when dipped in cool water for 15 to 20 seconds.

Cayenne. Hot red pepper works well, both externally and internally. Sprinkle about 1/4 teaspoon in your socks or gloves to warm up your extremities and take about 1/4 teaspoon 1 to 3 times a day (1 size 00 gelatin capsule) to improve your circulation.

Health Sandals. These are simple rubber sandals with tiny protrusions on the insole, which massage and stimulate your feet as you walk. You only need to wear them for about 10 minutes a day.

Vitamin E. This vitamin is excellent for improving blood flow to the hands and feet. Start with 1600 I.U. daily for 6 weeks. If there is no improvement, discontinue the dose. But if there is improvement, reduce the dose to 1400 I.U. for another 6 weeks and see if the improvement continues.

If it does, then reduce to 1200 I.U. for another 6 weeks. Whenever the positive effect begins to taper off, then you know you've just passed your maintenance dosage. For best results, continue that dosage daily, at least during the cold months. (For precautions concerning taking vitamin E, see chapter 5.)

Niacin (Vitamin B3). This is another member of the B complex, but in this case, it should be taken separately because when it's included in B complex pills, it is usually in the form of niacinamide. For circulation problems, niacin is specifically recommended. Take 100 mg. 3 times a day for 1 month. It will cause a hot flush within about 10 minutes. Don't be concerned; it will go away within about 15 minutes. This flush is part of the cure; it is caused by a dilation of blood vessels and increased blood flow to the face.

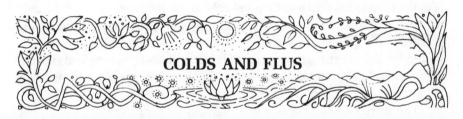

COLDS AND FLUS

A cold is rarely be attracted to a well-rested, relaxed, properly fed, and generally happy body. Colds have a particular affinity for overworked, tense, tired, poorly nourished, depressed bodies.

A cold is not altogether a bad thing. I've learned to see it as a friendly reminder that I've been overworking and neglecting my body. It puts me to bed where I can drink nourishing teas and juices and allow my subconscious dream mind to take over for awhile so my rational mind can rest.

I used to think I was clever. A cold would come, and I would drink my teas and take my vitamins and continue working. I never got sick enough to go to bed, but the cold would hang on for weeks.

Now I can feel when I'm starting to get overworked; I can predict when the cold symptoms will start to set in. It may be a slight sore throat or sniffles or just a feeling of exhaustion. If I listen to the signals, I'll go directly to bed. I might just sleep in for a morning, or I might take the whole day off and set myself free from the workaholic bandwagon. If I do this, I simply don't get sick.

Some people just can't give themselves permission to have a good cry—so they'll have a head cold instead.

I've grouped colds and flus together because most of the remedies are the same. They are both viral infections, and both enter through the respiratory tract, but a common cold tends to stay in the respiratory area. Influenza invades the respiratory tract and then spreads to the rest of the body. When there is abdominal pain, it is probably a stomach or intestinal flu, which is covered on page 197.

Prevention

If your body is starting to send you warning signals, and you simply cannot take the time to have yourself a good cold at the moment, you may be able to meet your body half-way. By using any of the following procedures, together with getting more rest, a good diet, and enough exercise, you should be able to strengthen your body's self-defense system and prevent a full-blown cold. But do yourself a favor and take a day off as soon as possible.

These are the most popular natural methods for preventing a cold, but they must be taken at the very first signs of a cold or flu: a little mucus, a slightly sore throat, a cough, or a sneeze. If you wait a day or two, "just to make sure," it will probably be too late.

Vitamin C. Some people take vitamin C every day, in varying quantities, and have reported a significant reduction in colds. People taking vitamin C at the earliest symptoms report that either the colds do not occur or they only last 2 to 3 days, and they're very mild.

Dr. Linus Pauling suggests between 250 and 5000 mg. per day as a maintenance dosage to prevent colds. The amount varies so widely because some people need more than others. At the *first symptoms* of a cold or flu, he suggests taking 500 to 1000 mg. every hour for several hours. *If the symptoms persist*, take 500 to 2000 mg. every 2 hours (or at least 4 times a day). Vitamin C is water soluble and passes out in your urine, so it should be taken frequently. If you get diarrhea, reduce the dosage. See chapter 5 for more information and precautions concerning taking large doses of vitamin C.

Animals—except for humans and apes—don't catch colds. We are practically the only animals that don't manufacture our own vitamin C. When other animals are infected by viruses, they respond immediately by increasing the rate of vitamin C manufactured in their livers.

During an infection, our metabolic rate increases, which causes vitamin C to be consumed faster than normal, so our need for this vitamin increases. If we take 1000 mg. of vitamin C when we have a cold, it can raise our white blood count. In this way, we mobilize our body's self-defense system, and we actively fight off the infection, rather than just suppress the symptoms.

Garlic. Garlic—especially organic garlic —is reputed to have antibiotic properties. Garlic and onions both contain allyl, an essential volatile oil that is rich in sulfur. At the first symptoms of a cold, take 1 or 2 cloves of raw garlic 2 or 3 times a day, until the symptoms are gone—and then for 2 or 3 more days.

You can chop it up and add it to an oil-and-vinegar salad dressing, or crush it and add it to the butter on your toast. It's good mixed with yogurt and grated cucumber. Or you can add it to chicken soup after the soup is cooked. Some people just chew it raw, or chop it up and swallow it down with water or tea.

Chopped garlic can be applied to the feet at night (a good remedy for infants). Apply vegetable oil to the feet first to prevent burning. Use 1/2 clove per foot. Wrap with gauze and then put on socks. By morning, you'll be able to smell the garlic on the breath.

As an antidote to the garlic smell, you can eat raw parsley. Kyolic is an odorless garlic that is becoming popular. Garlic capsules seem to be less potent than raw garlic for preventing colds and flus. The following tea tastes good, even to small children and to people who don't savor the taste or smell of garlic.

Note: Some people are allergic to garlic and respond by developing a stomachache or gas. Yogurt or acidophilus will give relief. But I'd suggest that you use another remedy if garlic affects you this way.

Recipe: Garlic and Lemon Tea. Bring 1 cup water to a boil. Cut 1 small garlic clove (preferably an organic one) into tiny pieces. Place in a cup and crush with a spoon. Add the juice of 1/4 small lemon and 1 teaspoon peppermint leaves. Cover and let brew for 3 to 5 minutes. Use honey if desired.

Hot Apple Cider Vinegar and Honey Tea. This is a convenient remedy to use when you are traveling because the ingredients are available in most homes and restaurants. It tastes a bit like hot lemonade. It's also very effective for breaking up mucus after a cold sets in.

This remedy was popularized by Dr. D. C. Jarvis in his book, *Folk Medicine.* He credits the effects of cider vinegar and honey to their high potassium content. The need for potassium is at a maximum in children, who use it to build tissues. This may be one reason why children have many more colds than adults, and their colds tend to last about twice as long.

Bacteria need moisture to maintain themselves, and they get this moisture by taking it out of the body cells. If there is enough potassium in each cell, it will draw moisture from the bacteria and they will not survive. Apples are also high in potassium, so it may be true that "an apple a day keeps the doctor away."

Recipe: Cider Vinegar and Honey Tea. Bring 1 cup water to a boil and add 1 to 2 tablespoons apple cider vinegar and 1 to 2 tablespoons honey (preferably raw). Stir and drink 1 to 2 cups per day.

Treatment of Colds and Flu

If your body does catch that cold, here are some basic guidelines to follow.

1. Go to bed and get as much rest as possible. If you have been overworking, stop working entirely for at least a day, or until your body feels renewed.

2. Stop eating, or at least avoid milk and cheese, which are mucus-producing. You may want to eliminate grains and meat for the same reason. Fresh salads are good. Or go on an all-fruit diet. Or a vegetable juice fast. These foods will help your body to eliminate toxins and take the strain off your digestive system, which will give your body more strength for healing. However, if you have a strong craving for a particular food, it may be wise to eat it (provided that it's nutritious).

3. Drink lots of herb teas and fruit or vegetable juices.

4. Wash your hands, particularly when you are sick, and especially before preparing or eating food. When you cough or sneeze, just turn your head. These viruses dry out and die very quickly in the air. Don't cover your mouth, because the virus can live up to 3 hours on your hands.

Sage, Garlic, and Lemon Tea. This tea is extremely effective for upper respiratory problems. It's good for coughs, congestion of the sinuses and lungs, as an expectorant (to raise phlegm), and for fevers (to induce sweating). It has also been used to ward off the flu, or to get rid of it quickly.

Garden sage can be purchased in any grocery or herb store. It's usually available as leaf sage or as ground sage. The leaf sage is most palatable for tea.

Recipe: Sage, Garlic, and Lemon Tea. Bring 6 cups water to a boil and pour over 2 heaping tablespoons sage leaves, 2 finely chopped garlic cloves (preferably organic), 1/2 lemon (juice and pulp), and honey (preferably raw) to taste. Steep for 5 minutes.

For best results, fast, and drink the tea while it's hot, at least 1 cup per hour. Stay in bed with plenty of blankets and sweat. Your temperature may go up temporarily, but this is a good sign if you are also sweating.

Tea for Colds. If you are willing to make a complex tea, the following will nourish your body, build up your immune system, help to eliminate toxins, and alleviate your symptoms. Use all of these herbs, or choose the ones that are appropriate to your condition based on the symptoms they alleviate. If any of these herbs are not available, just leave them out—or substitute another herb. You can add other herbs or garlic to this tea, or change the proportions. Herbs can be mixed together quite safely. The only herbs I don't mix together are comfrey and chamomile, because chamomile is reputed to destroy the allantoin in comfrey.

The echinacea root is good for blood cleansing, infections, sore throat, and swollen glands. The dandelion root is for detoxification and liver cleansing. Blackberry root cures diarrhea and sore throat. Comfrey acts as a cough suppressant and expectorant; it eases sore throats and strengthens the immune system. Coltsfoot treats coughs and headaches. Ephedra is given for chest congestion, sinus congestion, and sinus headache. Mullein is good for coughs, diarrhea, runny noses, and sore throats. Peppermint is good for dizziness, fever, headache, nausea, stomachache, and vomiting, as well as for flavor. Elder flowers are good for blood cleansing, diarrhea,

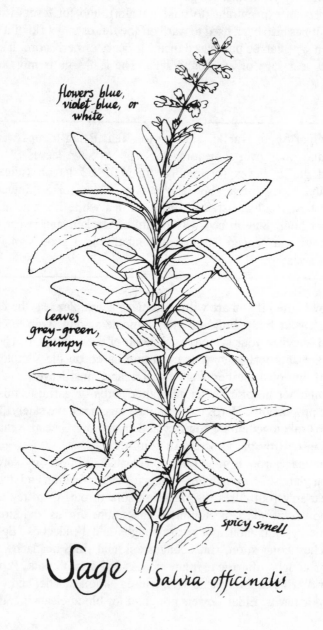

flowers blue,
violet-blue, or
white

leaves
grey-green,
bumpy

spicy smell

Sage *Salvia officinalis*

and fever. Catnip is given for nervousness, stomachache, and as an antidote for the stimulating effect of ephedra, as well as for flavor. Raw honey eases coughs and is soothing to mucus membranes and sore throats, while the lemon juice is good for coughs, as an expectorant, for sore throats, diarrhea, and blood cleansing.

Note: Please see the introduction to this chapter for cautions about comfrey. If you prefer, it can be eliminated from this tea. But since the proportion is so small, I believe it is safe for nonpregnant adults to use for up to 2 weeks.

There are various *Ephedra* species. It is also known as desert tea, Mormon tea, and ma huang. The latter is *Ephedra sinensis* or Chinese ephedra, which is more potent than American ephedra. So if you use ma huang, use about three-quarters as much.

Recipe: Cold Tea. Bring 10 cups water to a boil. Reduce to a simmer and then add 1 tablespoon echinacea root, 1 tablespoon dandelion root, and 1 tablespoon blackberry root. Simmer for 10 minutes and then add 1 tablespoon comfrey leaves, 1 to 2 tablespoons coltsfoot, 1 tablespoon ephedra, and 1 tablespoon mullein. Simmer for 10 minutes, and then remove the pot from the heat and add 2 to 3 tablespoons peppermint, 1 to 2 tablespoons elder flowers, and 1 tablespoon catnip. Cover the pot and steep for 5 to 10 minutes. Strain. Then add raw honey (to taste) and lemon juice and pulp, preferably organic (to taste). Brew for 5 minutes. Strain.

During a cold, drink as much as possible. People who have chronic colds can strengthen their resistance by drinking 1 or 2 cups every day.

Chicken Soup. Chicken soup has been raised to its proper status as a true remedy for colds by a study at the Mt. Sinai Hospital in Miami, Florida, which showed that chicken soup speeds the expulsion of germ-laden mucus from the nasal passages. They have actually isolated the chicken-soup factor.

Here's my mother's recipe (and it's a good one, whether you are sick or not).

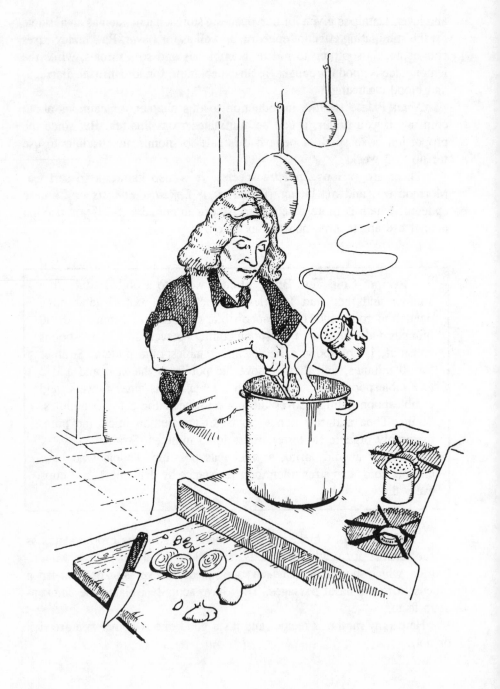

> **Recipe: Chicken Soup.** Wash 1 whole chicken in cold water. Place it in a pot and cover with water. Boil for 3 minutes, until it gets foamy. Skim off the foam. Chop 3 potatoes, 3 large carrots, 2 onions, 3 celery ribs with leaves and add to the soup along with the 3 garlic cloves, 1 tablespoon salt, 2 teaspoons onion salt, 2 teaspoons garlic salt, 1 teaspoon poultry seasoning, 1 teaspoon sage powder, 1 teaspoon celery salt, and 1/3 cup barley. Simmer for 2 to 3 hours, until the chicken begins to fall off the bones. Remove the chicken from the soup, allow to cool slightly, then strip the chicken off the bones, and return the meat to the soup. Eat as much as you like.

Chest Congestion

Dry air (lack of humidity) is a prime offender in aggravating this condition. Wood or gas stoves and radiators should have a pot of water on them to keep the air from drying out. If you suffer from frequent congestion, a cold mist humidifier is a good investment. Vaporizers can also be used, but the cold mist given off by humidifiers is more effective than the hot, moist steam given off by vaporizers.

Lung Tea. This tea is good for any cold, and particularly when there is congestion in the lungs. During a cold, drink as much as possible. People who have chronic congestion can strengthen their lungs by drinking 1 or 2 cups every day.

Note: Please see the introduction to this chapter for cautions about comfrey. If you prefer, it can be eliminated from this tea. But since the proportion is so small, I believe it is safe for nonpregnant adults to use for up to 2 weeks.

> **Recipe: Lung Tea.** Bring 6 cups water to a boil and add 1 tablespoon mullein, 1 tablespoon coltsfoot, and 1 tablespoon comfrey leaves. Simmer for 10 minutes, then add 1 tablespoon cornsilk (from Indian corn), 1 tablespoon lobelia, and 2 tablespoons peppermint. Brew for 5 minutes. Strain. Add as much honey as you want.

Eucalyptus Oil. This powerful aromatic oil is very penetrating, and it effectively breaks through congestion, making it easier to breathe. It can be purchased in any drugstore. Add 1 teaspoon of eucalyptus oil to the water in a cold mist humidifier or vaporizer. (The instructions often caution not to add anything to the water, but I've been doing this for years and have had no problems. Just wash the humidifier and clean the filter after each use.)

If you don't have a humidifier or a vaporizer, you can bring 2 cups water to a boil, remove the pot from the stove, and add 1/2 teaspoon eucalyptus oil. Put your head over the pot, cover your head with a towel, and inhale the fumes. Continue doing this for 5 to 10 minutes. You'll have to come up for air periodically.

If you have access to eucalyptus trees, use about 6 leaves and 6 seed pods in 2 cups of water. Simmer for 10 minutes, then strain and use as described above. This water can be saved and used again several times until it loses its potency.

Tiger Balm. This ointment is good to rub on the chest and upper back when you have chest congestion. It brings a sense of intense heat within 5 to 10 minutes after applying. It stimulates circulation and breaks up congestion. Tiger Balm is made from strong aromatic oils of camphor, menthol, peppermint, clove, and cajeput. (Cajeput is an oil from the East Indies that contains methyl salicylate.) There are 2 kinds of Tiger Balm: red and white. The red is considerably hotter than the white and works well on the back and chest. Keep Tiger Balm out of reach of children, because camphor is poisonous when taken internally. Keep away from eyes and mucous membranes, because it causes a burning sensation. (To avoid accidentally rubbing my eyes with a finger that has Tiger Balm on it, I use the fourth or fifth finger of my left hand to apply it.)

Tiger Balm is made in China and sold in many stores where Chinese items are found, as well as many herb and health food stores. It comes in small and large vials.

White Flower Oil. This oil is also from China, and it is similar to Tiger Balm, though it is even more penetrating. White Flower Oil is made with strong aromatic oils of menthol crystal, wintergreen, eucalyptus, camphor, and lavender. Apply as needed.

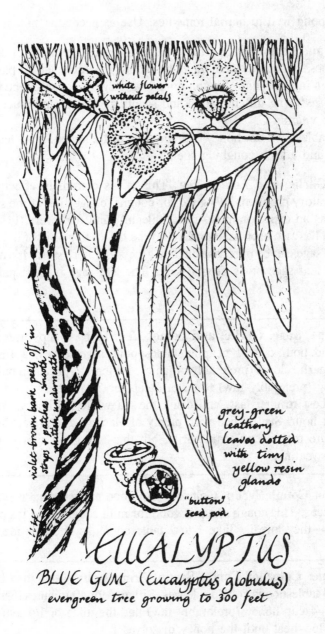

white flower
without petals

violet-brown bark peel off in strips + patches - smooth + whitish underneath

grey-green
leathery
leaves dotted
with tiny
yellow resin
glands

"button"
seed pod

EUCALYPTUS
BLUE GUM (Eucalyptus globulus)
evergreen tree growing to 300 feet

Coughs

Coughs respond well to herbal remedies. Use as needed.

Honey and Lemon Juice. This is the most popular remedy for coughs. Honey soothes the mucous membranes by coating the throat and air passages. It is also high in potassium. Lemon juice is astringent; it causes the tissues to contract, reducing inflammation and swelling. It also cuts mucus, and it is high in vitamin C.

Mix 1 tablespoon raw honey with the juice of 1/2 lemon. Sip 1 teaspoon every hour and after a coughing spell.

Sage, Garlic, and Lemon Tea. This tea is extremely effective for upper respiratory problems. It's good for coughs, congestion of the sinuses and lungs, as an expectorant (to raise phlegm), and for fevers (to induce sweating). It has also been used to ward off the flu, or to get rid of it quickly.

Garden sage can be purchased in any grocery or herb store. It's usually available as leaf sage or as ground sage. The leaf sage is most palatable for tea.

Recipe: Sage, Garlic, and Lemon Tea. Bring 6 cups water to a boil and pour over 2 heaping tablespoons sage leaves, 2 finely chopped garlic cloves (preferably organic), 1/2 lemon (juice and pulp), and honey (preferably raw) to taste. Steep for 5 minutes.

For best results, fast, and drink the tea while it's hot, at least 1 cup per hour. Stay in bed with plenty of blankets and sweat. Your temperature may go up temporarily, but this is a good sign if you are also sweating.

Coltsfoot Cough Syrup. Coltsfoot is a good expectorant; it helps to bring up mucus. This cough syrup is good for mild coughs, and it's perfect for children—they love it. Take 1 to 2 tablespoons as often as needed.

Recipe: Coltsfoot Cough Syrup. Bring 1 cup water to a boil and add 3 tablespoons coltsfoot leaves. Simmer for 10 minutes. Strain and add 1/4 cup honey (preferably raw) and the juice of 1/4 lemon. Place on low heat until the honey dissolves.

Cayenne. I use this effectively for coughs that won't respond to anything else. It works quickly to loosen the phlegm. It has expectorant, astringent, and antispasmodic properties. Take 1/4 teaspoon of cayenne as often as needed. You can take it in a 00 capsule, or sprinkle it on your salad or in your soup. Or put the cayenne on the tip of a butter knife and drop it on the back of your tongue and quickly wash it down with liquid (there aren't many taste buds on the back of the tongue).

For a real hearty remedy, mix 1/4 cup whiskey, 1/4 cup fresh lemon juice, and 1/4 teaspoon cayenne. Drink it down, go to bed with lots of blankets, and sweat.

Nasal Congestion

The mucous membranes of the nose may become inflamed due to a cold. The symptoms include a "runny" or "stuffed-up" nose, sneezing, and "runny" eyes. Try to avoid commercial nose drops or sprays, which relieve by constricting the blood vessels and shrink the swollen mucous membranes. After about 3 days, the blood vessels lose their ability to constrict and the symptoms are worse than ever.

It is helpful to keep the mucus thin so that the sinus passages and the eustachian tubes don't get plugged. Do this by drinking lots of fluids and by using a cold mist humidifier.

For dry nasal passages, apply one of the following with a cotton swab: vitamin E oil (just open a capsule of vitamin E with a pin and squeeze out the oil), vegetable oil (any kind will do, as long as the smell is agreeable), or calendula ointment (available in health food stores; see Index: Calendula ointment). Dry air (lack of humidity) is a prime offender in aggravating this condition. Wood or gas stoves and radiators should have a pot of water on them to keep the air from drying out. If you suffer from frequent congestion, a cold mist humidifier is a good investment. Vaporizers, which give off hot, moist steam, can also be used, but cold mist humidifiers are more effective.

Eucalyptus Oil. See page 70 for a discussion of this penetrating oil.

Tiger Balm. To open nasal passages and facilitate breathing, it's good to apply white Tiger Balm to the area between the eyebrows, and to the temples and earlobes. Be careful to avoid the sensitive mucous membranes inside your nose and avoid the lips, because it brings a sense of intense heat within 5 to 10 minutes after applying.

Ephedra Tea. This is wonderful for loosening mucus. You may find that ephedra is stimulating and will speed up your heart.

There are various *Ephedra* species. It's also known as desert tea, Mormon tea, and ma huang. The latter is *Ephedra sinensis* or Chinese ephedra, and it's more potent than American ephedra. So if you use ma huang, use three-quarters as much for small children; see precautions under Asthma and Bronchitis, page 34.

Recipe: Ephedra Tea. Bring 2 cups water to a boil and add 2 teaspoons granulated ephedra or a small handful of ephedra twigs. Simmer for 10 minutes. Drink 1/2 cup 3 or 4 times a day, or as needed. If prepared for children under 10, give only half as much.

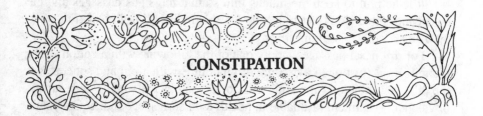

CONSTIPATION

The symptoms of constipation are uncomfortable bowel movements with small, hard stools, bowel movements so infrequent that you feel uncomfortable, or a sense of incomplete evacuation. Elimination is a vital life function, and when your plumbing is clogged, all sorts of other illnesses can follow. If you aren't satisfied with your elimination, take it as a sign that you are not eating and living properly.

Constipation is also a common complaint during pregnancy. During pregnancy, your body produces high levels of progesterone which cause the relaxation of your smooth muscles. This affects your intestines by reducing their motility. As the fetus in your belly grows larger, your stomach and intestines are displaced and compressed. Peristalsis (contractions of the intestines which aid digestion) is slowed down and food remains in your stomach longer. Your stomach secretes less hydrochloric acid and pepsin, which are important in the breakdown of proteins. All of these factors combine to slow down digestion, which leads to constipation.

Constipation can also be caused by food allergies. For example, many people are allergic to wheat, but they don't know it. They don't break out in hives and nothing dramatic happens when they eat wheat. But when they eliminate or minimize this one food, they find that within a few days their feces become soft.

Before looking for remedies, examine the following guidelines and see if your diet and lifestyle are conducive to proper elimination.

Water. Constipation is often caused by insufficient fluid so the stools get hard and dry. Try to drink 8 or more cups of fluid a day (2 quarts). Coffee, black tea, and beer do not count because these are diuretics and cause you to lose fluid. Juices and herb teas are good, but clean, pure water is best.

Tension. This is a major cause of constipation, and reducing tension will probably be necessary before the problem will be eliminated. A good therapist or a friend may be a big help. Jogging or running or some other vigorous activity may be a good way to blow off steam. See also the section on Nervous Tension.

Exercise/Yoga. Exercise is vital for good health and good elimination. Yoga and other exercises that make use of the abdominal muscles sometimes stimulate peristaltic action. A good abdominal massage may also be helpful.

Pay Attention to Your Body. When you have the urge to go to the bathroom, take advantage of it. Don't put it off. Don't strain; try to relax. Set aside about 10 minutes a day for this vital activity. Some people like to do this at the same time each day—after breakfast, for example. Some people find that squatting is helpful. Others like to put their feet on a stool in front of the toilet.

Eat Slowly and Chew Thoroughly. Many people find this makes a big difference. Chewing produces saliva, which aids digestion.

Raw Greens. Eat plenty of greens, especially raw ones—they put roughage in your diet.

Dietary Remedies

If you are still having difficulties, here are some remedies you can try (in order of their popularity).

Bran. This is by far the most popular remedy for constipation. Many long-standing, chronic cases respond to it beautifully. It's a food, so it works gently, without irritating the colon. Bran has a remarkable capacity to absorb moisture, so when it's taken with plenty of liquid, it swells up and forms a soft mass that passes easily through the intestines. Raw or crude bran can be purchased in health food stores, and is preferable to most packaged commercial bran cereals which contain less than one-third the fiber content and are often heavily sweetened. Remember to drink plenty of liquid (1 to 2 cups) at the same time, and drink more throughout the day.

People report taking anywhere from 2 tablespoons to 1 cup of bran per day. Many like to mix it with orange juice or cereal or bake it in muffins.

Recipe: Bran Muffins. Preheat the oven to 375° F. Combine and mix 2 cups wheat flour, 1-1/2 cups bran, 2 tablespoons brown sugar (optional), 1/4 teaspoon salt, 1/4 teaspoon baking powder (without aluminum), and 1-1/4 teaspoons baking soda.

In separate bowl, beat together 2 cups buttermilk, 1 beaten egg, 1/3 cup molasses, and 1/4 cup vegetable oil.

Combine the contents of both bowls and mix with a few strokes, then add 1 cup raisins. Mix just until all the dry ingredients are wet.

Pour the batter into greased tins. For normal-size muffins, fill the tins to two-thirds full. For huge muffins, fill almost to the top. Bake for 25 minutes. Makes about 12 normal-sized muffins.

Prunes or Prune Juice. This traditional remedy for constipation is easily obtained and often works quite well. Use as needed. Start with 1 cup of juice, or 1/2 cup of stewed prunes per day, and increase until you get the desired result. Children under 10 should have half as much.

To make stewed prunes, barely cover dried prunes with water, add a touch of lemon juice, and simmer for about 20 minutes. Add other dried fruits, such as raisins and apricots, if you like.

All-Fruit Diet. Many people like to cleanse their colon by eating only fruit, fruit juices, and water for 1 to 5 days. Some like to do this 1 day a week. Others do it whenever they feel congested.

Molasses. This is a safe, mild laxative. It can be added to yogurt, milk, or cereal, or put on pancakes. Adults should take 1 to 2 tablespoons per day, and children should have 1 to 2 teaspoons.

Yogurt or Acidophilus. This will help to stimulate your intestinal bacteria to do a better job of breaking down your food. Eat as much as you like: at least 1 to 2 tablespoons of yogurt or 1 to 2 teaspoons of acidophilus each day.

Recipe: Bran-Yo-Lax. This combines the laxative properties of yogurt, bran, molasses, and dried fruit. Feel free to increase the proportions of any of the ingredients. Mix together 4 tablespoons plain yogurt with 2 tablespoons raw bran, 1 teaspoon molasses, and 1 teaspoon raisins. This should always be taken with at least 1 cup of liquid (water, herb tea, fruit juice). Children under 10 may need only half as much bran and molasses.

Warm Water and Lemon Juice. Mix the juice of 1/2 to 1 lemon with 1 cup warm water and drink this before bedtime, or in the morning, at least 30 minutes before breakfast.

Liver Flush. Take 1 teaspoon to 1 tablespoon olive oil and 1/2 to 1 1/2 lemons before bedtime.

Raw Flaxseed Meal. Grind raw flaxseed in a blender or coffee grinder and add 2 tablespoons flax meal to approximately 1 cup water, juice, herb tea, or cereal.

Orange Water. Take 2 sips of orange-charged water before each meal. (For more information on color-charged water, see Index: Color healing.)

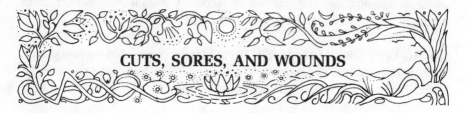

CUTS, SORES, AND WOUNDS

Large cuts may leave scars unless they're stitched, but they cannot be stitched after 6 to 8 hours. Be sure to see a doctor soon if the wound is serious.

Bleeding

Some bleeding is good, because it cleanses the wound. But excessive bleeding can be dangerous. Most cuts or wounds will stop bleeding if pressure is applied directly to the wound, or to the artery that feeds into the wound. Apply pressure to cuts by first covering with sterile gauze, and then applying even pressure. Vitamin E can be applied to the cut to promote normal clotting. Calendula ointment also helps to stop bleeding. And cayenne can be sprinkled on wounds to stop bleeding.

Cleaning the Wound

If you haven't had a tetanus shot in the last 8 years, consider getting a booster immediately. Tetanus cannot grow in the presence of air, so puncture wounds are the most likely place for them to grow. However, tetanus has been known to grow in other minor wounds. If you haven't had an up-to-date tetanus shot, it's particularly important to thoroughly disinfect the wound.

In any case, remove all dirt and foreign materials and clean with soap and water. If the wound hasn't been bleeding, encourage it to bleed by squeezing the flesh. This is nature's way of cleansing. Sometimes a bath or a soak is the easiest way to accomplish this. Then use one of the following disinfectants.

Apple Cider Vinegar. Dab on undiluted, or soak with 1 part apple cider vinegar and 8 parts hot water for 10 minutes.

Golden Seal and Myrrh. Bring 1 quart of water to a boil and sprinkle in 1 teaspoon powdered golden seal and 1 teaspoon powdered myrrh. Cover and steep for 5 minutes, then strain, and wait until the temperature is tolerable. Do a hot soak for 10 minutes or sprinkle the powders, mixed in equal parts, over the wound.

To make a paste of golden seal and myrrh, use equal parts of each powder and mix with a little water. Apply the paste directly to the wound. It should be washed off once or twice a day and the wound should be exposed to the air for about an hour. Then fresh golden seal and myrrh can be applied again. (Some people use plain golden seal, usually with good results, but the combination of both herbs is more consistently effective.)

Hydrogen Peroxide. If the above is not available, you may have this standard disinfectant. (If you like, this can be applied first, then the golden seal and myrrh can be sprinkled on.)

Note: Do *not* use alcohol, tincture of iodine, or merthiolate directly in a wound; it will only damage the flesh and slow the healing.

Ointments and Poultices

Comfrey. This fine herb is the most popular remedy for all kinds of wounds. It causes them to heal quickly and draws out infections. Comfrey promotes rapid cell proliferation, which enables skin to grow back together quickly.

Comfrey can be prepared in many ways. Usually the fresh leaves are used. I like to prepare a comfrey paste which combines the healing properties of comfrey, vitamin E, and raw honey. Such a paste can also be kept through the winter, when fresh leaves aren't available, and shared with people who don't have their own plants.

To make a comfrey paste, combine equal parts of olive oil and raw honey in a blender and process. Then remove the center of the top of the blender and gradually add washed and chopped fresh comfrey leaves. Add enough to reach the desired thickness. Then add a bit of melted beeswax to harden and preserve it. The paste can then be put into containers. I usually carry one small container in my purse, and keep the rest in the refrigerator. Apply once or twice a day, as needed. Various similar comfrey ointments are also available in health food stores.

To make a comfrey poultice, you'll need access to a fresh comfrey plant. Just cut off a leaf or two, macerate with a mortar and pestle or clean rock in a bowl. This brings out the juices and makes the leaves less prickly. Apply directly to the wound. Then wrap with clean gauze or cloth. Change this poultice once or twice a day.

To do a comfrey soak, make a strong comfrey tea. For each cup of boiling water, add 1/4 cup tightly packed chopped fresh comfrey leaves or 3 tablespoons of dried leaves. Simmer for 10 minutes. Then strain. Allow to cool to a comfortable temperature. Immerse the wound in the solution, and soak for 10 to 15 minutes.

Vitamin E. The oil from this vitamin is a popular ointment for all kinds of wounds, causing them to clot and heal quickly. To apply, puncture a capsule of vitamin E oil with a pin, and squeeze directly onto the wound. For best results, use vitamin E from natural sources (see chapter 5 on Vitamins and Minerals for more information). Repeat 1 to 3 times a day. Some people prefer to buy vitamin E cream, which contains high concentrations of the vitamin. Vitamin E should also be taken internally, 100 to 800 I.U. daily, until the wound has healed.

Vitamin E has a remarkable ability to prevent scarring, because scar tissue forms in the absence of sufficient oxygen. Blood carries oxygen to all the tissues of the body, and when there is a wound, the tiny blood capillaries are cut and the oxygen can't get to the cells. Vitamin E is helpful because it makes maximum use of the oxygen in the blood.

Plantain. This remarkable herb grows almost everywhere, and makes an excellent poultice for cuts and wounds. It has strong drawing properties, and therefore helps prevent or relieve infections. If you are healthy, the leaf can be chewed. If not, macerate it as described under comfrey, above. Apply the pulp directly to the injured area, just enough to cover it. For

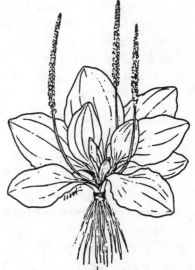

PLANTAIN
(BROADLEAF or COMMON)
Plantago major
a common "weed" of moist lawns and
waste places - naturalized from Europe

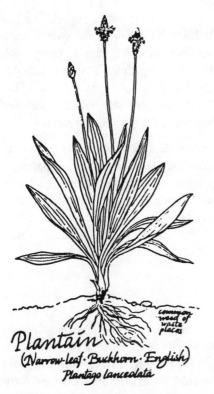

common
weed of
waste
places

Plantain
(Narrow-leaf · Buckhorn · English)
Plantago lanceolata

minor wounds, just allow it to stay on the skin for a few minutes, then resume your activities and it will fall off by itself. For more serious wounds, put a bandage over the plantain, and change it once a day. Plantain grows almost everywhere, but it doesn't grow in cold climates during the winter, so make a paste, as described under comfrey above, using plantain leaves instead of comfrey, or equal parts comfrey, plantain, and burdock leaves (since burdock is also healing to the skin). This is an all-purpose paste that's useful for a wide range of skin problems, especially if there is any sign of an infection.

Aloe Vera Gel. This is soothing for cuts and wounds. Cut off the tip of one of the lower leaves of an aloe plant, peel back the skin of the leaf, and apply the gel directly on the wound. The plants are available from some florists. The bottled gel is not as effective.

Calendula Ointment. Made from calendula, or pot marigold, this is a great remedy for cuts and wounds. It helps to relieve pain quickly and speeds healing. Calendula cerate comes in a tube, it's easy to carry with you, it's reasonably priced, and it lasts for a long time. This is a popular remedy with naturopaths and homeopaths. Just apply as needed. This ointment is available at some health food and herb stores, and wherever naturopathic and homeopathic remedies are sold (see Resources).

Raw Honey. This makes a fine ointment, and it is usually available. Honey has antiseptic properties—it kills bacteria. This may be partially explained by the presence of formic, malic, and lactic acids. It attracts and absorbs moisture, which may also account for its ability to destroy bacteria and germs, since they require moisture in order to live. Some doctors in England use honey for infections instead of antibiotics. Perhaps the nutritive properties help the tissues to regenerate and heal.

Bandaging

Exposure to air helps promote healing. But if it is not possible to keep the wound clean, it is better to bandage it, at least until it forms a scab. However, be sure that the bandages are clean and dry, or else they may do more harm than good. Flaps of skin should be left on because they form a natural dressing, unless they can't be cleaned properly, in which case they should be cut off carefully.

Long cuts are liable to leave scars unless the edges are pulled together. This is usually accomplished by stitches, but if the cut is on an area of the body that doesn't get too much stress, or doesn't get wet (unlike the drooling chin of a baby), you can purchase "steri-strips" or "butterfly" band-aids from the drug store. First be sure the wound is clean. Then join the edges of the wound so that it looks more or less the way you'll want it to look when it's healed. Then apply the steri-strips going perpendicular to the cut, approximately 1 every 1/4 inch.

Infected Sores

Soak the sores 2 or 3 times a day, using a disinfectant, such as apple cider vinegar or golden seal and myrrh (see above) in water as hot as can be tolerated, for 10 to 15 minutes. Then apply comfrey or plantain as directed above. Expose to the air for at least 1 hour each day.

If the infection does not improve after 24 hours, consult a medical worker. Sometimes neosporin or bacitracin (no prescription needed) or some other antibiotic ointment may be advisable. (See also the section on Staph Infections.)

When to See a Medical Worker

If blood is pumping vigorously from the wound, this indicates possible damage to a major blood vessel. Apply firm pressure to the vessel, above the site of the wound, until help can be found.

If there is fat protruding from the wound (especially on the chin); or if the wound is deep, and it is on the head or trunk or hands, consult a medical worker. Any large wound may require stitches. It will have to be treated within 8 hours because germs can grow in the wound, and stitching would trap them inside. Numbness, tingling, or weakness in the affected limb could indicate possible damage to major nerves.

If an infection develops and does not respond to home treatment (symptoms of infection are fever, pus, extensive redness, and swelling), or if there is foreign material that you can't remove in the wound, consult a medical worker.

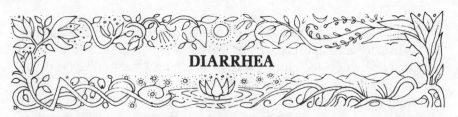

DIARRHEA

Diarrhea is present when there are frequent watery stools. There are many causes. It is the body's natural form of elimination. Diarrhea can be a healthy phenomenon if it lasts for just a day or two. But if it goes on for a long time, you will be losing valuable nutrients. The most common causes of this complaint are eating too fast, eating too much (especially late in the day), and nervous tension. Some people, particularly vegetarians, may suffer from perpetually loose stools due to insufficient protein. Frances Moore Lappé's *Diet for a Small Planet* is an excellent book on how to get maximum protein from nonmeat sources.

If you live in the country and have frequent diarrhea, consider testing your water for bacterial contamination from sewage or manure run-off. If you suspect that the water may be the problem, 10 drops of iodine in a gallon of water will kill many bacteria. Boiling water for 20 minutes kills most germs.

Some people get diarrhea as an allergic reaction to milk. This is especially common among black people and many third-world people. They lack the enzyme lactase, which breaks down lactose (milk sugar). In children, frequent diarrhea may be a sign of a food allergy. Antibiotics can cause diarrhea. Food poisoning can cause diarrhea.

You tend to get diarrhea when you are scared, or when you can't hold on to things.

Remember that an occasional bout of diarrhea may be your body's way of cleansing. Fasting is a way of furthering this process. Otherwise, wait at least 6 hours before you try to stop the diarrhea. Give your body a chance to do its work first. If you try one or two of these remedies and don't get results within 48 hours, consult your health care provider.

Fasting. Try fasting for 24 to 36 hours. Only drink liquids and avoid milk or milk products, sweetened fruit juices, and honey. Drink clean, pure water if you can. Get plenty of fluids. Fasting is recommended because it allows your system to cleanse itself. An infection often breaks off the brush border on the villae of the small intestines, and then your body can't absorb carbohydrates. If you fast for 36 hours, you allow the brush border to grow back. Babies and small children often fast spontaneously; they should be allowed to do this. However, if a child really wants to eat, offer grains (barley and brown rice are good) and use one of the other remedies.

For serious cases of diarrhea, the fasting should be accompanied by just a tablespoon of apple juice every 15 minutes. This quenches the thirst and keeps the small intestines from becoming bloated with too much fluid. If this amount of fluid is tolerated, it can be gradually increased. Add 1 tablespoon every 2 doses. When the normal *number* of bowel movements have occurred for at least 16 hours, try eating a mild grain, such as barley or brown rice (for small children, grind the rice in a blender and cook with 4 parts water). Avoid milk. If the usual number of bowel movements continue for the next 12 hours, a normal diet can be resumed gradually.

Cinnamon and Cayenne Tea. Cinnamon is an intestinal astringent that is good for gas. It has an amazingly quick effect on most cases of diarrhea. It will bind very quickly, so it's beneficial in stopping the loss of fluids and important nutrients. This is my favorite remedy for diarrhea, but if you feel that the body needs a cleansing, don't use this remedy.

Recipe: Cinnamon and Cayenne Tea. Bring 2 cups water to a boil and add 1/4 teaspoon cinnamon and a dash of cayenne. Simmer for 20 minutes. Cool and strain.

Take 2 tablespoons every hour, as needed. For babies and children under 6, use 1/8 teaspoon cinnamon, avoid the cayenne, and give doses of 1 to 2 tablespoons. This remedy usually tightens the bowels immediately, so don't give more than necessary.

Cinnamon can be used in various other ways; for example, sprinkled on apple sauce or toast.

Apple Sauce. Pectin occurs naturally in apples. It is used in jam-making to thicken the jam, and it does the same for the feces. Applesauce sprinkled with cinnamon is a painless medicine. Or you can take an apple, peel it (the peel can be difficult to digest), and grate it. There is more pectin in the part of the apple that is closest to the skin. Kaopectate, a common drug for diarrhea, contains pectin.

Acidophilus or Yogurt. Sometimes diarrhea occurs when the intestinal bacteria have been weakened. Lactobacillus acidophilus is a beneficial bacteria that grows naturally in your intestines and elsewhere. Lactobacillus bulgaricus is a similar bacteria which is found in yogurt.

The bacteria count in your intestines can be multiplied by taking acidophilus or yogurt. Some forms of yogurt have added acidophilus. Acidophilus is sold in liquid and tablet form. Health food stores usually carry both. Most drugstores carry acidophilus tablets. For diarrhea, take 1 to 2 tablespoons of the liquid, or 1 to 3 tablets, 3 or 4 times per day. Or eat about 4 tablespoons (1/4 cup) of plain yogurt every 2 to 3 hours while awake.

Human mother's milk is an original source of acidophilus, so you could make your own acidophilus yogurt by adding 1 tablespoon of mother's milk per cup of warm milk, to start an acidophilus colony growing in it. Mother's milk yogurt is an excellent remedy for chronic digestive disorders.

Bran. Bran is good for diarrhea because it works like a sponge, soaking up excess liquid. Raw or crude bran can be purchased in health food stores. It's preferable to packaged commercial bran cereals which contain less than one-third the fiber content and are heavily sweetened. Remember to drink plenty of liquid (1 to 2 cups) at the same time, and drink more throughout the day.

People report taking anywhere from 2 tablespoons to 1 cup of bran per day. Many like to mix it with orange juice or cereal or bake it in muffins. (See Index for recipes.)

Preventing Dehydration. Good juices to give when diarrhea occurs are apple, grape, and cranberry. For babies under 1 year, mix with an equal amount of water.

Good teas (taken separately or in combination) to take with diarrhea are blackberry (use the leaf or the root or the green berries) or strawberry leaf tea. Nourishing teas (to keep the strength up) include comfrey (leaf or root), nettle, red clover, peppermint, and/or ginger (fresh grated is best).

When to Call a Medical Worker

If diarrhea lasts longer than 48 hours, consult your health care provider. The main danger with diarrhea is dehydration, which most commonly occurs when there is diarrhea *and* vomiting. Dehydration can be fatal, particularly in infants.

If there is also pain on urination, diarrhea could be caused by a kidney or bladder infection.

If there is extremely fast or labored breathing, or blueness in the lips or fingertips, pneumonia could be the cause of diarrhea or vomiting.

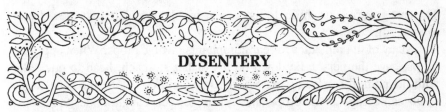

DYSENTERY

Dysentery is usually characterized by "the runs," which is an unusually fluid discharge from the bowels. Also there may be fever, stomach cramps, and spasms of involuntary straining to evacuate with little result. The stool is often mixed with pus and mucus and may be streaked with blood. Dysentery usually occurs in unsanitary and crowded conditions. In Mexico it is called "tourista," because it is a common affliction of tourists.

When you have dysentery, there is real danger of getting seriously dehydrated (loss of water and lowered blood sugar). Dysentery leaches out many nutrients from the body, especially niacin and magnesium. It can be especially dangerous to infants, children, the elderly, and others in a weakened condition.

Dysentery can cause attacks of diarrhea over a long period of time. If untreated, complications involving the liver and lungs may result. The following are possible ways to *prevent*, not to cure, dysentery. See a doctor if you suspect you have contracted dysentery.

Garlic. When traveling, eat a clove or two of raw garlic a day. (See the Index: Garlic, for suggestions on palatable ways to consume raw garlic).

Acidophilus. While traveling, take a tablet of acidophilus 2 or 3 times a day.

Vitamin C. While traveling, take 1000 mg. of vitamin C 2 or 3 times a day. (See chapter 5 for more information on vitamin C.)

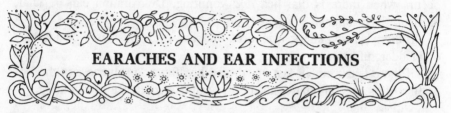

EARACHES AND EAR INFECTIONS

The ears govern your ability to listen. Ear problems tend to indicate a desire to shut someone out.

Many of the remedies for ear complaints involve drops. When applying drops, have the person lie down on his or her stomach, head to one side, with the painful ear facing up. Slowly drip the drops along the canal wall, so air can escape as the drops enter. If the air gets caught under the drops, the drops won't get into the ear. If this happens, pull down on the earlobe.

Wax in Ears/Ears Plugged

If there is a feeling of fullness in the ears, or if there seems to be some loss of hearing, use a pen light or flashlight and try to look inside the ear.

Ear wax is normally self-draining. It filters dust and keeps the ears clean. Well-intentioned people who frequently use cotton-tipped swabs for cleaning the ears can actually cause the wax to become impacted against the eardrum. One doctor says, "Never put anything smaller than an elbow in your ear." It is best to leave the wax alone, unless it becomes uncomfortable, or crusty, or turns black, or causes some loss of hearing.

For these problems, the following suggestions are helpful.

Garlic Oil. Garlic oil capsules are sold in most health food stores. Puncture 1 or 2 of these caps with a pin and squeeze the oil into a teaspoon. Hold the teaspoon over a match or candle and heat until it is warm, but not hot. Use a dropper to insert the oil into the ear as described above. The person should lie this way for 10 to 15 minutes, then turn the head to the other side, with a paper towel or tissue under the ear, to allow the ear to drain. Place a half-filled hot water bottle or a heating pad set on medium under the tissue to soften the wax and enable it to drain freely. Have the person remain in this position for at least 15 more minutes.

Another method is to peel a clove of garlic, cut it in half, dip it in oil, and insert it just behind the tragus (the flap of skin in front). Do not attempt to push the garlic deep into the ear. Leave it overnight—but remove it sooner if it becomes irritating.

Olive Oil. Use a teaspoonful of olive oil as described above. Plain vegetable oil has also been used effectively. Some people prefer to plug the ear with a small piece of cotton and leave the oil in overnight.

Earaches

Serous otitis media is a nonbacterial ear infection. Usually there is a feeling of fullness in the ear or some temporary loss of hearing. These symptoms can be treated at home unless they last for more than 10 days.

Swimmer's Ear (Otitis externa) is characterized by itching and burning in the ears. Wiggling the earlobe may cause pain. This infection of the external ear canal often occurs after swimming or getting the ear full of water. It can develop into a more serious bacterial infection.

A minor earache often responds well to the following remedies.

Sweet Oil. This old-fashioned remedy works by reversing the permeability of the eardrum and drawing out the infection. It is used by some doctors. Place 1/4 teaspoon sugar and 1/4 teaspoon olive or vegetable oil in a teaspoon. Heat over a candle or match until until warm. Place in the ear with a dropper as described above, then plug with a small piece of cotton. Remove after 12 hours. Repeat 12 hours later if necessary.

Garlic Oil. Open 1 or 2 capsules of garlic oil with a pin. Heat and apply as with the sweet oil. Alternatively, you can peel a clove of garlic, cut it in half, dip it in oil, and insert it just behind the tragus (the flap of skin in front). Do not attempt to push the garlic deep into the ear. Leave it overnight—but remove it sooner if it becomes irritating.

Mullein Oil. This is inserted into the ear with a dropper. Mullein oil may be found in some herb and health food stores, or it can be ordered from the Standard Homeopathic Company (see Resources). Or you can make it yourself: gather the yellow mullein flowers and pack them tightly into a glass mason (canning) jar. Then leave the jar in the sun for 2 days. The flowers should exude oil. Pour off the oil.

Middle Ear Infections (*Otitis Media*)

This is an inflammation of the middle ear, and it is quite common among children. It usually begins with a cold, followed by congestion and swelling of the mucous membrane lining of the middle ear. Then the cavity fills from the discharge, and the eardrum may bulge. The child may feel pain, or heat, or a fullness in the ear and may experience a dullness of hearing, which later changes to severe pain with increased loss of hearing and a feeling of general illness. Earaches can be detected in infants and very young children when the child's hand frequently goes to the ear, or if the child rolls his or her head from side to side, or if the child cries when you press the front or back of the ear. If the discharge becomes pussy, the eardrum may rupture, which can result in a loss of hearing. However, the eardrum will usually repair itself, either partially or completely.

Many children are plagued by chronic middle ear infections. Louise Hay suggest that this problem often occurs in families where there is a great deal of shouting and arguing. The common medical treatment is antibiotics and decongestants, which wage war within the body, leaving a person feeling very weak and lethargic. An excellent alternative is acupressure, which should be combined with the decongestant ephedra syrup. Mullein oil is also effective for otitis media, and echinacea is useful for any infection.

Acupressure. A child's skin is relatively thin, so children are extremely receptive to acupressure. Many adults find this method effective also, though some require the insertion of acupuncture needles at the same points. I've treated many children with this method, and taught their parents how to do it, and none have had to use antibiotics for middle ear infections since. To prevent recurrence, begin treatment at the first sign of pain, and new infections will never develop. One child had congenitally small eustachian tubes and this remedy prevented his having to have plastic tubes inserted.

Children are usually receptive to this method, particularly when they realize that they can stop using medicines, and some can actually feel their ears draining during or just after the first treatment. Press the ball of your fingertip gently and repeatedly at the points listed below. If there is pain, then be more gentle. When treating a small child, it often feels like there is so little being done that it can't possibly have any effect, and yet it does.

If there are older children present, I like to demonstrate on them, since little ones often imitate big kids, and it won't do any harm to a healthy child. I also like to demonstrate on the parents. Children usually enjoy

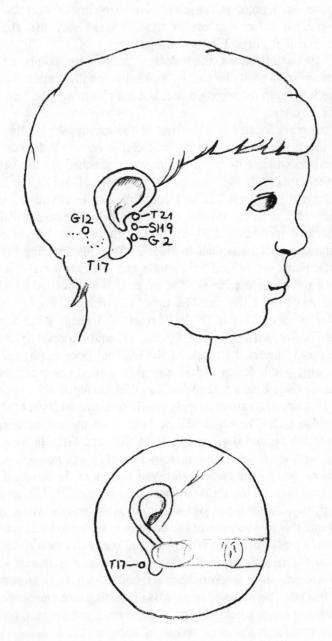

counting games, so I ask them to count with me while I give the treatment. Twenty taps at each point is sufficient. I take plenty of time for these rituals to establish an atmosphere of trust. I make sure that the child understands that if it hurts, I'll be more gentle.

For middle ear infections, the following acupressure points are used. These points are most easily located by looking at the illustration. No harm will be done if you tap the wrong place, but the results will be best if you get the right location.

T21 is the point located just in front of the ear, level with the top of the tragus (the fleshy flap of skin in front of the center of the ear hole), in the depression which fills when the jaws are clenched. In the language of acupuncture, this is Triple Warmer 21, Erh Men, Door of the Ear.

Si19 is located just below T21, in front of the ear, level with the middle of the tragus. This is Small Intestine 10, T'ing Kung, Listening Palace.

G2 is located just below Si19, in front of the ear, slightly below the bottom of the tragus. This is Gall Bladder 2, Ting Jui, Hearing Meeting.

T17 is the point just behind the earlobe and in front of and level with the bottom of the mastoid process. The mastoid is an inverted triangular-shaped bone just behind the ear. The tip of the triangle is level with the bottom of the earlobe. This is Triple Warmer 17, I Feng, Wind Screen.

G12 can be located by feeling for the mastoid process. If you run your finger up the inverted triangle of the mastoid bone, along the back (posterior) edge, you'll feel a little depression a short distance from the bottom. This is Gall Bladder 12, Wan Ku, Whispering Bowl.

On the first day of treatment, apply gentle pressure with your fingertip at T21, G2, and G12. The child will probably feel the ear draining immediately. On the second day, tap gently at Si19 and G12. *If there is no improvement within 48 hours, the therapy probably will not be effective, and it would be best to use the conventional treatment.* However, if there is improvement, then on the third day, return to points T21, G2, and G12. By the fourth day, most of the symptoms probably will be gone, but be sure to *continue this treatment until the hearing is fully restored to normal.* This may take a week or more. When you feel ready to discontinue treatment, give just 2 treatments in the last week because it is best to stop gradually. Have a medical worker check the child's ears to make sure they are entirely healed. There should be no loss of hearing (compare both sides with the ticking of a watch held at varying distances from the ear), no fever, no aches, no ringing in the ears, and no dizziness.

For best results, this treatment should be combined with ephedra syrup.

Ephedra Syrup. Ephedra is a natural stimulant and can increase the heartbeat considerably. In this syrup it is combined with catnip, which is a sedative. You may want to avoid using the syrup just before bedtime. Ephedra is also known as Desert Tea or Mormon Tea. Chinese ephedra, or Ma Huang, is considerably stronger than American ephedra, so use only three-quarters as much.

Dose: babies take 3 or 4 eyedroppers; small children take 1 to 2 teaspoons; children over 10 take 3 to 4 teaspoons. The dosage can be repeated 3 or 4 times a day. This is a very potent syrup and should be used with care.

Recipe: Ephedra Syrup. Bring 2 cups water to a boil and add 3 heaping tablespoons granulated ephedra. Simmer for 20 minutes. Remove from the heat and add 3 tablespoons catnip. Steep for 5 minutes.

Echinacea. This herb is excellent for infections because it promotes rapid healing and is also antiseptic. The easiest way to take echinacea is to buy the tincture and take 10 drops in 1/4 cup water or juice, 4 times a day. Alternatively, you can take the powdered herb in 00 caps. Take 1 capsule 3 or 4 times a day. Or take the syrup as directed below.

Recipe: Echinacea Syrup. Bring 1 1/2 cups water to a boil. Add 4 tablespoons dried echinacea root (or 1/2 cup fresh root); simmer for 20 minutes. Remove from the heat. Add 1/4 cup fresh peppermint. Steep for 5 minutes. Strain and add honey to taste (about 1/4 cup). Adults should take 1 to 2 tablespoons of syrup 3 times a day until the infection subsides. The dose for infants under 3 is 1/4 teaspoon 3 times a day. Children under 10 should take 1 teaspoon 3 times a day. If this remedy causes stomach pain, discontinue.

Mullein Oil. This is inserted into the ear with a dropper. Mullein oil may be found in some herb and health food stores, or it can be ordered from the Standard Homeopathic Company (see Resources). Or you can make it yourself: gather the yellow mullein flowers and pack them tightly into a glass mason (canning) jar. Then leave the jar in the sun for 2 days. The flowers should exude oil. Pour off the oil.

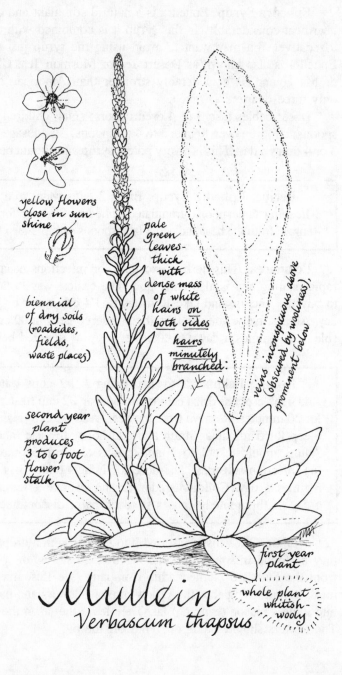

yellow flowers
close in sun-
shine

pale
green
leaves-
thick
with
dense mass
of white
hairs on
both sides

hairs
minutely
branched:

biennial
of dry soils
(roadsides,
fields,
waste places)

second year
plant
produces
3 to 6 foot
flower
stalk

veins inconspicuous above
(obscured by wooliness),
prominent below

first year
plant

whole plant
whitish-
wooly

Mullein
Verbascum thapsus

Itchy Ears

Itchy ears could be a symptom of Swimmer's Ear (see above). Here are some simple remedies that have been effective. See page 88 for instructions on applying ear drops.

Vitamin A. Puncture a vitamin A capsule with a pin and squeeze the contents of 1 capsule into each ear. Repeat daily as needed.

Isopropyl Alcohol. Use a dropper and fill the ear with 100 percent isopropyl alcohol for 20 to 30 seconds. Then let it drain out. It dries out the ear immediately.

Apple Cider Vinegar. Use a dropper and fill the ear with apple cider vinegar for 20 to 30 seconds. Then let it drain out.

Fungus or Scabs Behind the Ear

This generally can be prevented by washing behind the ears. But if you get a scab-like growth behind the ears, wash it well and then apply a comfrey paste (see Index) or salve. Wash it off the next day, and repeat if necessary.

When to Call a Medical Worker

If the ear is very painful, or if the ache does not respond to treatment within a few hours, consult a medical worker. An earache may be the sign of a middle ear infection, which can be quite serious.

If there is blood or pus coming out of the ear, if an earache follows a cold, if hearing loss continues for more than 10 days, if it is very painful and the pain lasts over an hour (even if it seems to go away after that), or if the temperature is over 102° F., see a medical worker. If you can't touch your chin to your chest without pain, this could be a sign of meningitis. Dizziness or trouble with balance could indicate inner ear problems.

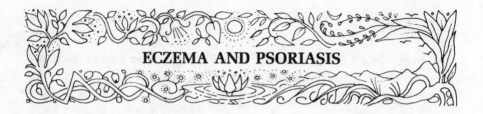

ECZEMA AND PSORIASIS

Eczema and psoriasis are both skin rashes. Eczema is characterized by itching, swelling, blistering, oozing, and scaling of the skin. It is a common allergic reaction in children, but it also occurs in adults—usually on the face, neck, and folds of the elbows and knees. Psoriasis is a chronic, recurrent ski disease marked by bright red patches covered with silvery scales. It most commonly appears on the knees, elbows, and scalp.

These diseases tend to occur to people who are thin-skinned, easily hurt. Louise Hay associates psoriasis with a fear of being hurt, feeling dead to yourself, refusing to accept your own feelings.

The following remedies have been effective. After 2 weeks, the condition should be significantly improved. Continue to drink at least 1 cup of cranberry juice a day, preventatively. Repeat the whole regime if a new outbreak occurs. But don't use cod liver oil for more than 2 weeks at a time, and wait at least 2 weeks before using it again.

Halve the recommended dose for children under 10.

Cod Liver Oil. Take 2 tablespoons a day.

Raw Sesame Oil. Take 1 teaspoon raw sesame oil a day. It can be used on salads, but don't cook with it.

Cranberry Juice. Drink 3 cups of cranberry juice a day. Any brand is okay.

Aloe Vera. Apply as needed. For more information, see Index: Aloe vera.

Comfrey Ointment. Apply as needed. For more information, see Index: Comfrey ointment.

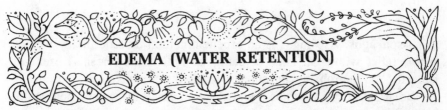

EDEMA (WATER RETENTION)

Edema occurs when abnormal amounts of fluid pass out of the blood vessels and into the tissue spaces (the interstitial or intercellular spaces). This can be caused by a low protein diet. Birth control pills (which contain estrogen) are another cause of water retention. High estrogen levels just before menstruation can cause sodium retention, which results in edema.

Vitamin B6. This vitamin is well-known for its ability to eliminate water retention. Vitamin B6 sets up a balance of sodium and potassium in the body, which regulates the body fluids. Try taking 10 to 50 mg. per day. Menstruating women may need as much as 100 mg. per day. Experiment to find the best dosage for yourself. Begin with 10 mg. and then increase by 10 mg. more each day until you achieve the desired effect. Use the whole vitamin B complex. (See chapter 5 for more information on B vitamins.)

Vitamin C. This is an effective, natural diuretic. Take at least 500 mg. 3 times a day. (See chapter 5 for more information on taking large doses of vitamin C.)

Water. Many people have found that drinking lots of water helps relieve edema. Perhaps it works by washing out the salt and stimulating the kidneys.

Potassium. This mineral is important for maintaining a good water balance in the body. Also, potassium aids your body in handling salt (sodium). Sodium tends to pull fluid outside of the cells, whereas potassium draws fluid into the cells. Diuretics wash out many minerals, including potassium. Potassium deficiency is usually characterized by lack of energy and muscular weakness. See chapter 5 on Vitamins and Minerals for foods rich in potassium and supplement your diet as needed.

Calcium or Calcium/Magnesium Supplements. These are particularly useful for premenstrual edema.

Asparagus. Asparagus is an excellent natural diuretic. Many women report relief within an hour of eating several stalks—fresh, frozen, or canned. You'll probably be able to smell the asparagus in your urine. Be sure to take extra vitamins B and C and minerals (especially potassium) about 2 hours after using any diuretic (including beer and coffee) because these wash out your water-soluble vitamins and minerals.

Localized Edema

Edema or swelling in just one part of the body (as with a sprain) can often be relieved by elevation of the part and application of cold to the area. When edema occurs as part of an allergic reaction (as with a bee sting), a doctor should be consulted, because if the swelling becomes severe, the respiratory passages could close off and you could suffocate.

EYE COMPLAINTS

The eyes are likely to give you trouble when you are reluctant to look at the world around you, when you try to hide the truth from yourself, and when you hold back your tears.

Object or Gunk in the Eyes

Usually, the twisted corner of a piece of tissue paper or a handkerchief will do the trick. Some people like to use an eyeglass with water or boric acid solution. But if these simple methods do not cleanse the eye, here is another home remedy.

Chia Seed. Chia seeds are available in most health food stores. They are small (about the size of sesame seeds) and become mucilaginous when moist, thereby attracting objects to themselves. Moisten one seed (you can put it in your mouth for a moment—saliva is probably the best moistening agent for this purpose), then pull out the lower eyelid and drop in the seed. It can be left in from 5 minutes to 12 hours. The seed has the ability to draw any excess mucus, gook, or unwanted material to itself. When it has served its purpose, or if it becomes uncomfortable, just coax it to the inner corner of the eye (the corner of a tissue works nicely) where it can be easily removed. Flax seed is often used the same way, but it is much bigger and can be uncomfortable.

Infected Oil Follicle in the Eyelid

Chia seeds, used as directed above, may also be successful. Or try lightly brushing the follicle with a dry cotton swab each day.

When to See the Doctor

If the eye was struck forcefully with a small particle of metal, the particle could have penetrated the eyeball. Cover each eye separately and test your vision. If your sight does not seem normal, get it checked. If the foreign body remains in the eye, it may be trapped behind the upper lid. Finally, if there is blood in the eye, or if the eye is painful, consult a doctor.

Irritated Eyes (Conjunctivitis, Pinkeye)

The eyes become sore, red, irritated, or gooey when the thin membrane (the conjunctiva) that lines the eye and eyelid and gets inflamed. This may be due to an irritant in the air (such as smog or smoke), an allergy (such as hay fever), a virus (such as herpes), or bacterial infection (such as gonorrheal conjunctivitis). Pinkeye is highly contagious.

If this happens with a baby under 2 months old, see a doctor immediately to be sure it isn't gonorrhea or inclusion conjunctivitis.

The following remedies can be applied 3 or more times a day with an eye dropper or with a ball of cotton over the closed eye.

Chamomile Eyewash. This is a traditional remedy that has worked well for many people. Cover 2 teaspoons chamomile flowers (German chamomile is best) with 1/4 cup boiling water. Cover and steep for 3 to 5 minutes. Strain through a cheesecloth (I put it through a small strainer first; then I empty the strainer, line it with a piece of double-folded cheesecloth, and strain again).

Eyebright Rinse. Cover 1/4 teaspoon of eyebright (herb) and cover with 1/4 cup boiling water. Steep for 15 minutes, then strain through a cheesecloth as directed above.

When to Call a Medical Worker

If the problem doesn't clear up after a few days of home treatment, if the discharge gets thicker, if there is pain in the eyes, if there is a decreased ability to see, if there is pain from bright lights, or if the discharge is like pus (thick or green or yellow-green), call a medical worker.

Tired, Strained Eyes

Tibetan Eye Chart. Some people have strengthened their eyes (though not necessarily improved their vision) by using this chart, which resembles a large black snowflake. The idea is to follow the outline of the pattern with your eyes to give the eyes a wide range of exercise. It takes only a minute or two a day. The chart, with complete instructions for its use, can be ordered from the Herbal Holding Company (see Resources).

Palming. Rub your palms together to warm them, then cup them over your closed eyes for several minutes. The warmth and exclusion of light are very soothing. It helps to rest your elbows on a table or put a pillow on your lap. Do this at least once a day.

Azurite. This is a lovely blue stone. It can be placed over each eye when the eyes are strained—as when you have been driving or using a computer for too long. Put one stone (preferably a polished or tumbled stone) on each closed eyelid, near the corners toward the nose. After 15 to 30 minutes, your eyes should feel rested. This can be combined with crystal energization (see Index).

Sty on the Eye

A sty resembles a pimple. It is an inflammation of one or more of the sebaceous glands of the eyelid. Like a boil, it occurs when bacteria gain entrance into the skin and cause the formation of pus. Hot compresses applied for 15 minutes 4 times a day help to localize the infection and promote drainage.

Black Tea Bag. The tannic acid in black tea draws out the infection. Moisten the tea bag with hot water, squeeze out the excess water, and apply to the sty; the tea bag should be as hot as possible without burning. Keep dunking the bag in hot water to keep it hot. You'll probably feel immediate relief. The skin of the eyelid may peel a bit, as with a sunburn, but there should be no discomfort.

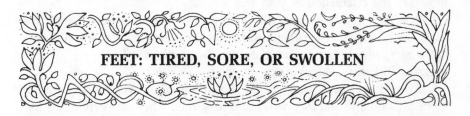

FEET: TIRED, SORE, OR SWOLLEN

Your feet carry you forward in life. Problems with the feet often indicate a reluctance to go forward, or confusion about what direction to take. When your feet are tired, sore, or swollen, consider the following.

Appropriate Shoes. Good shoes go far in keeping the foot free of aches and pains. High heels or even normal heels lock your calf muscles into a contracted position, as if you were constantly walking downhill.

Tight shoes squeeze your toes, causing discomfort and tension throughout your body.

Try to find shoes that have a good inner padding, that give you support, that don't pinch your feet, and that feel comfortable to wear all day. If your feet are uncomfortable, your nerves will be constantly on edge. If you find a comfortable shoe, you'll be doing your feet, legs, back, and nerves a big favor.

Birkenstock, a German manufacturer of sandals and shoes, makes shoes that are specially designed to promote the health of your feet and legs. Recently, other manufacturers have begun to copy the Birkenstock design, resulting in a wider variety of shoes with similar features.

If you place your feet in the sand, they leave a footprint with natural contours under the arch and the toes. The foot itself remains level, with the heel and the ball of the foot on the same plane. When the foot remains in this natural position, it gives the greatest relaxation to your feet, legs, and even your buttocks and back. Birkenstocks provide a foot bed that is contoured to the natural shape of your foot. They provide ample room for your toes to spread without being pinched. The soles of these shoes are made of lightweight cork, which absorbs shock and provides natural support. Most Birkenstocks are open in the back, like clogs, forcing the foot to make a slight squeezing motion with each step to keep the shoe on. This constant squeezing massages your foot and calf muscles, which increases the circulation in your feet and legs.

Ironically, many people who suffer from cold feet have found that Birkenstock sandals (worn with warm socks) keep their feet warm during the winter, whereas heavy boots do not. Boots pinch off your circulation, whereas Birkenstocks contribute to good circulation.

Birkenstocks (and most similar shoes) are expensive, but they tend to be of high quality and they will last a long time when properly cared for. Look in the Yellow Pages of your telephone directory under shoes, and then under Birkenstock. Birkenstocks are available in most large cities.

Foot Baths. It's wonderfully soothing to soak your feet. It refreshes your whole body. Preparing a foot bath is one of the nicest things you can do for someone who has been on their feet all day. Children love to do it, too. In fact, when one person gets their feet soaking, the whole family usually wants to get in on it.

Begin by finding a basin or pot large enough to hold at least 1 foot with water up to the ankle. Then fill the basin with water so you'll know how much water you will need. Pour this amount of water into a big pot and bring to a boil. Then add either comfrey or epsom salts as directed below. When the preparation is ready, fill the basin about one-quarter full of cold water, then add some of the preparation. Keep the rest in a covered pot so it will stay hot. When the preparation in the basin is comfortably hot, put your feet in. When it begins to cool, add more of the hot preparation.

Comfrey Foot Bath. Add 2 handfuls of fresh or 1 handful of dried comfrey leaves per gallon of boiling water and simmer for 10 minutes. Strain and use as directed above.

Epsom Salts. This is actually a form of magnesium, which is very soothing. It is available in any drugstore. Add 1/4 cup of epsom salts per gallon of hot water and use as directed above.

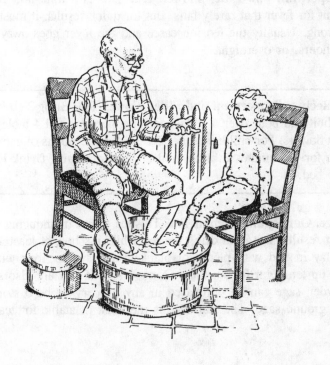

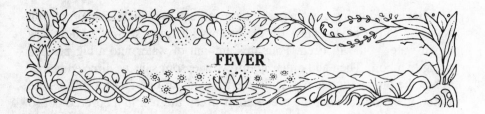

FEVER

There is a fever if the temperature (which should not be taken immediately after extreme physical activity) is 100° F. (38° C.) or more by mouth. During a fever, take more than normal amounts of fluids, since the fever is literally burning up your body's moisture.

In an adult, any fever over 101° with a sore throat, or over 102° for 5 days, or in a child, over 103°, should be reported to a medical worker.

Avoid aspirin. There are natural methods for treating fevers which are very effective.

Peppermint and Elder Flower Tea. This is a time-honored herbal treatment for fever that rarely fails. But for quick results, it must be made very strong. Usually the tension eases and the fever goes away within a couple hours, or overnight.

Recipe: Peppermint and Elder Flower Tea. Bring 2 cups water to a boil and pour over 4 tablespoons peppermint and 4 tablespoons elder flowers. For children under 10, use 2 tablespoons of each herb. Steep for 15 minutes in a covered container. Strain. Drink hot and go to bed.

Sage, Garlic, and Lemon Tea. This tea works by inducing sweating. For best results, fast, and drink the tea while it's hot, at least 1 cup per hour. Stay in bed with plenty of blankets and sweat. Your temperature may go up temporarily, but this is a good sign if you are also sweating.

Garden sage can be purchased in any grocery or herb store as leaf sage or ground sage. The leaf sage is the most palatable for tea.

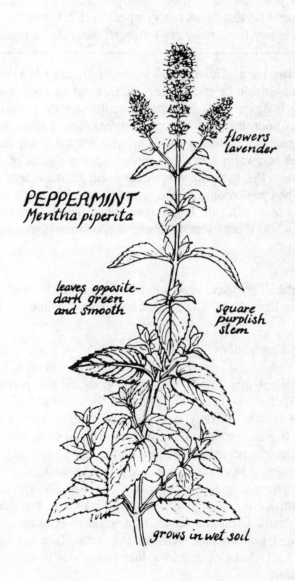

flowers
lavender

PEPPERMINT
Mentha piperita

leaves opposite-
dark green
and smooth

square
purplish
stem

grows in wet soil

> **Recipe: Sage, Garlic, and Lemon Tea.** Bring 6 cups water to a boil and pour over 2 heaping tablespoons sage leaves, 2 finely chopped garlic cloves (preferably organic), 1/2 lemon (juice and pulp), and honey (preferably raw) to taste. Steep for 5 minutes.

Cooling the Heat. This method is frequently used in hospitals. If a fever is uncomfortable or if it exceeds 102°, tepid or cool water can be used to bring it down. Start by running cool water on a washcloth and applying it to your forehead, temples, wrists, and hands. Repeat this every 5 minutes. If it doesn't seem to bring down the fever, then lie in a shallow tub of lukewarm water and sponge alternate parts of your body and extremities. The moisture evaporation will increase heat loss from your body. When you become chilled, get out of the tub, and wrap yourself in a blanket, but do not rub. Begin again when the chill passes. Do this in a warm (not hot) room, with no drafts. Discontinue if your temperature drops too quickly.

Blue Light. If you have access to a colored lamp, lie with your head under the blue light. This should reduce your fever within 10 minutes.

Treating Convulsions. A high fever of 105° of more may come on quickly with a child and may lead to seizures or convulsions. Convulsive involuntary spasms may involve the whole body or just part of it. The child gets stiff, clenches the jaw and fists, and the eyes roll back. The child may hold the breath, possibly turn blue, salivate, urinate, or defecate. Though very frightening to parents, such convulsions are not considered serious in children who are between 6 months and 4 years old. They can usually be prevented in children who are prone to having convulsions by beginning to reduce a fever whenever it goes above 101° (rectally 102°).

If a convulsion does occur, roll the child on his or her side to allow the saliva to drain. Clear the mouth of any saliva or vomit to facilitate breathing. Don't put anything between the teeth. Take off clothes and sponge with cool cloths or put in a lukewarm bath to bring down the body temperature.

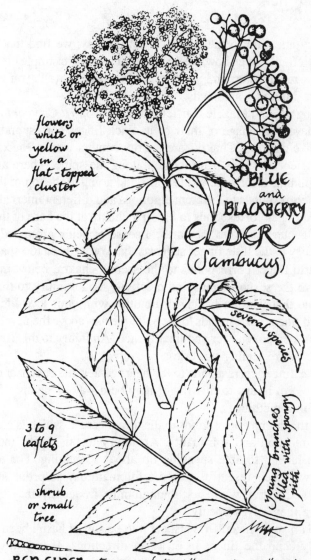

flowers white or yellow in a flat-topped cluster

BLUE and BLACKBERRY ELDER (*Sambucus*)

several species

young branches filled with spongy pith

3 to 9 leaflets

shrub or small tree

RED ELDER - stronger, can be toxic; flowers not generally used

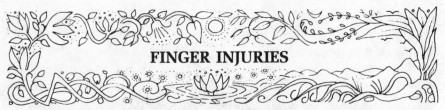

FINGER INJURIES

When we pay attention to the language of the body, we find that injuries to the hands often reflect how we handle things. For example, if you are upset about a relationship and you are not handling it well, you may find that you have injured your hands.

According to Laeh Maggie Garfield, author of *Spirit Companions*, even the fingers have a language of their own. Each finger corresponds to one of the first five chakras. Chakras are energy centers which—according to the ancient science of yoga—are located along the spine. There are seven chakras, beginning at the base of the spine and going to the top of the head. Each chakra corresponds to different emotions and different internal organs.

The little finger corresponds to the first chakra at the base of the spine. This energy center relates to the earth; a sense of being grounded, stable, centered. Injury to the little finger suggests that you've been too spaced out.

The fourth finger corresponds to the second chakra, below the navel. This relates to the sexual organs and creativity, so an injury to this finger could indicate that you are having difficulties with your love life.

The third finger corresponds to the solar plexus (above the navel), which relates to your personal power and intelligence. An injury to this finger may indicate that you're feeling powerless or stupid.

The index finger corresponds to the heart center, the center of compassion and love. An injury to this finger may be a way of saying "I haven't the heart" for something.

Finally, the thumb corresponds to the throat center, which is concerned with communication and spirituality. An injury to this finger may occur when you're having trouble speaking up about something. For example, a carpenter who feels resentful toward a foreman may be prone to a blow to the thumb. Children who suck their thumbs frequently may be afraid of expressing themselves openly.

If you slam your finger, first inspect it to be sure it hasn't been broken. Try to gently bend the finger in different directions. If any direction is extremely painful, then consult a medical worker. If ice is available, apply it immediately, for at least 10 minutes, to reduce the swelling.

Poultice. After removing the ice, apply the macerated leaves of plantain or the pulp of garlic or onion to the nail for 3 minutes or more. Remove at once if it becomes more painful. Plantain is a common weed, found on most unsprayed lawns. If you are healthy, the simplest way to macerate the leaves is to wash and then chew them (saliva also has healing properties and plantain doesn't taste bad). Alternatively, any of these substances can be chopped fine and mashed with a mortar and pestle, or a wooden spoon in a cup.

Pressure. Firmly squeeze the same finger of the opposite hand. This is a folk remedy practiced in both North America and China. Chinese medicine advises that when you cannot treat an area of the body because the pain is too intense, you should treat the corresponding place on the opposite side. The Chinese use the concept of yin and yang to explain why pressure relieves pain: Yin and yang are opposite forces, and whenever anything is taken to its extreme, it will turn into its opposite, just as day follows night. Similarly pain is yang, and by applying more yang in the form of pressure, we are forcing the pain to turn into its opposite, yin, which disperses the pain and causes relaxation.

Blood Blister Under Nail

If the fingernail or toenail gets hit hard, it may turn red in one spot under the nail. This is a blood blister, and it is usually extremely painful, especially if the blister swells and builds up pressure under the nail. If you are feeling extreme pain and pressure, the following technique will release the pressure, and it will usually save the nail. It is recommended by many doctors.

Paper Clip. Straighten a paper clip, heat it on a constant light source (a stove or candle) until it is red hot, and then apply very firmly to the nail, over the red spot. You may have to re-heat and re-apply the paper clip 2 or 3 times, until a small hole opens in the nail, which will allow the blood to drain out.

It may sound unpleasant, but if this isn't done, the whole joint of the digit may swell and turn blue, pressure will build up, the pain will be excruciating, and the nail will probably fall off. To prevent infection, put a couple drops of apple cider vinegar on a band-aid and cover the nail.

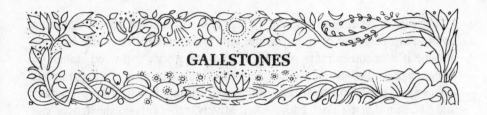

GALLSTONES

The gallbladder is a small saclike organ located below the liver, where bile is stored. Sometimes calculus in the gallbladder will form into stone-like masses. This is most common in overweight women and in men and women over the age of 35. If you have gallstones, you are probably suffering from severe gas pains and sharp pains under the right rib cage where the gallbladder is located. At first, these pains seem directly related to eating certin foods, especially fatty foods, but after a while it may seem like you can't eat anything without feeling pain.

Gallstones tend to occur when things or people or situations in your life are galling you. They are also associated with not getting enough pleasure in life.

Though gallstones are considered a very serious disease, curable only by the surgical removal of the gallbladder, it is one of the easiest ailments to cure naturally. I have known over a hundred people who have used this technique, many of whom were already scheduled for surgery— and I only know one case where surgery was still needed (and no harm was done by having used this remedy).

This wonderful remedy comes from a book called *Herbal Cures of Duodenal Ulcer and Gall Stones* by Frank Roberts. The complete program takes about 24 hours, though there are rare cases that go on for longer. You will need 1 pint (2 cups) of pure olive oil and 4 or 5 medium-size lemons. If fresh lemons are not available, use bottled lemon juice. Try to find a brand of olive oil that is reasonably palatable.

Before beginning the treatment, do not eat any solid food after your midday meal. Wait until about 2 hours before your normal bedtime and then begin the treatment. I recommend timing it with a good television program to divert your attention from the difficult task at hand.

Every 15 minutes for the next 2 hours, drink 1/4 cup (4 tablespoons) of olive oil followed by 1 tablespoon of lemon juice. The lemon juice acts as a chaser, helping you to hold down the olive oil and making a better taste in your mouth. The last dose or two is usually the most difficult to take, and it may help to mix the lemon juice with the olive oil and take them both at once.

It is essential that *all* of the olive oil be taken each time, and that the entire pint should be taken on the same evening—even if vomiting occurs. The oil softens the stones and lubricates the ducts so that the stones will move easily through the ducts and come out in the feces.

After taking the full dose, you can go directly to bed. You will probably sleep through the night, though you may wake up either to pass stool or to vomit. During the 24 to 48 hours after taking the remedy, people pass at least 50 and up to 150 green rubbery "stones" varying in size from a split pea to a ping-pong ball. The passing of large stones is sometimes accompanied by a feeling of nausea or faintness or pain, but this passes very quickly. Nevertheless, I recommend having someone present to give you support if you need it.

Frank Roberts says that in 20 years, he has never seen a case that has not cleared completely within 6 months (and stones passed within 48 hours), provided that people took the full dosage. Some of these people had stones that were lodged in the gall duct. I only know of one case that might be called unsuccessful, where a woman passed sand (it literally looked exactly like sand) every day for 2 months, and she did feel considerably better, but she felt eager to be totally done with it and so she opted for surgery. Robert says that he has seen 2 cases of bilirubin stones, which were red like strawberries.

Most people like to save at least the larger stones, and many take pleasure in bringing them to their doctors. Since the stones usually float, the simplest way to do this is to get a pair of rubber gloves and a plastic spoon and fish them out of the toilet bowl. Rinse them and put them in a jar with a lid; the smell is not pleasant. After a couple of days, the stones will liquefy into an oily liquid.

Do not plan to do anything during the day and night following your treatment because you will probably feel quite weak and may need to make frequent and sudden trips to the bathroom. However, after 24 to 48 hours, you will probably feel better than you have felt in a long time.

For the next month, take the following herbal formula to alleviate the inflammation of the gallbladder and gall duct.

> **Recipe: Gallbladder Formula.** Using powdered herbs, combine
> the following:
> 1 tablespoon Oregon grape root
> 1 teaspoon wild yam
> 1 teaspoon cramp bark
> 1 teaspoon fennel seed
> 1 teaspoon ginger
> 1 teaspoon catnip
> 1 teaspoon peppermint
> Fill 00 capsules with the mixture and take 2 caps with warm water
> before each meal for the next month. Try to take them 15 to 20 minutes
> before each meal.

Also take 1 capsule of lecithin before each meal. The lecithin will help to break down fats, and the herbs will soothe the inflammation and prevent gas. During this month, be careful to avoid fried, fatty, greasy, and spicy foods, as well as pastries and cakes. Minimize your use of oils of all kinds in order to give your gall bladder a rest. After 1 month, you can begin to gradually bring oils back into your diet, but it is just as well to avoid most of these foods if you want a healthy diet. Nevertheless, within 6 months, you should be able to eat normally without discomfort.

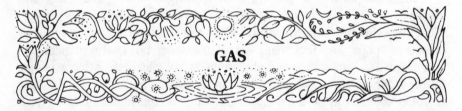

GAS

Gas occurs when air or other gases accumulate and distend the stomach or intestines, causing discomfort or belching or a discharge of "wind" from the rectum. The most common causes of gas are eating too fast, not chewing properly, eating when nervous or not hungry, eating when overtired, eating just before bedtime, and overeating. Gas may also be part of an allergic reaction to certain foods, such as milk or garlic.

Gas is also common during pregnancy, when the intestines are being squeezed by the growing fetus. Also the increased production of progesterone during pregnancy relaxes the smooth muscles, including the uterus, blood vessels, intestines, stomach, and cardiac sphincter, causing them to become quite lax. Progesterone slows down the peristalsis (contractions) of the intestines and stomach so that food remains longer in the stomach, where it tends to ferment and produce gas.

Certain foods are more likely to cause gas: onions, garlic, cabbage, turnips, large amounts of brewer's yeast, and beans—the worst offender. Various methods are mentioned to prevent gas from beans, though none seem to be reliable. You might try 1) soaking the beans overnight and discarding the soaking water, or 2) soaking the beans overnight with a piece of fresh papaya or meat tenderizer made from papaya (active ingredient papain) and cook in the same water, or 3) bring the beans and water to a gentle boil, then discard the water and cook in fresh water, or 4) add ginger or summer savory or fennel seeds to the beans while they cook, or 5) cook in a pressure cooker.

Certain food combinations are considered gas-producing. This is explained by the fact that different enzymes are required to digest different kinds of foods and they work less effectively when forced to work at the same time. The following combinations are often cited as causing gas: fruits and vegetables, cereals and acid fruits, cherries and dairy products, miso and fruit. It is suggested that you wait 2 hours between foods that make poor combinations.

If gas occurs, the following remedies are effective.

Aromatic Seeds. It is a common practice among East Indians to finish a meal by chewing a few pinches of aromatic seeds. This helps prevent gas. Caraway seeds, fennel seeds, anise seeds, or licorice root can be chewed (1/4 to 1/2 teaspoon at a time) or made into tea (use 1 teaspoon per cup and simmer for 10 minutes).

Mint Tea. A popular carminative, meaning it prevents gas. Any kind of mint can be used: peppermint, spearmint, catnip, etc.

Recipe: Mint Tea. Cover 1 teaspoon of mint with 1 cup boiling water and steep for 5 minutes.

Slippery Elm. This is an extremely effective remedy, even for very serious cases of gas. This herb is usually taken in powdered form, in 00 capsules. For best results, swallow the capsules with warm water or tea, which will help them to dissolve. Or prepare slippery elm tea, which tastes okay but has a peculiar, mucilaginous texture, which some people find disagreeable. Slippery elm is also mildly laxative, tending to make the stools somewhat slippery.

Recipe: Slippery Elm Tea. Bring 1 cup water to a boil and sprinkle in 1/2 teaspoon powdered slippery elm bark, or 1 teaspoon granulated or plain slippery elm bark. Simmer for 20 minutes. Strain. Drink 1 to 3 cups per day.

Yellow Fluorite. Fluorite is a gemstone that comes in many remarkable shapes and colors. Fluorite is good for the nerves, and the color yellow relates to the digestion. If your problem with gas was caused partly by nervous tension, place a yellow fluorite octahedron (double pyramid) over the painful area and lie down and breathe deeply for at least 5 minutes. This can be combined with crystal energization (see Index).

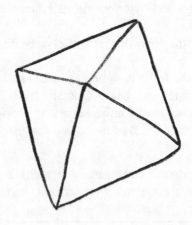

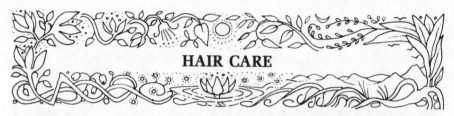

HAIR CARE

Your shampoo is probably the most important part of your hair care. Be wary of the new "natural" shampoos that have a long list of chemicals in fine print on the back of the bottle. Health food stores carry many good shampoos. Try alternating 2 or 3 brands because they all take something out of your hair.

The following rinse can used in place of conditioners to remove the soap residues, maintain the acid pH of the hair, and leave your hair soft and shiny. Apple cider vinegar is the most popular hair rinse, though the vinegar makes you smell like a salad unless it is combined with sweet-smelling herbs and allowed to sit for about a week. Lemon juice (bottled or fresh) brings out blonde highlights, but it is not recommended for people with dry hair because it strips the oils from the hair.

To make a hair rinse, pour 2 tablespoons of cider vinegar or lemon juice in a quart jar. After you have shampooed your hair and rinsed it with clear water, add warm water to the jar and slowly pour over your hair, working it into your scalp. Do not rinse your hair again.

Rosemary will make your hair shiny. Pour 2 cups of boiling water over 2 tablespoons of fresh (preferred) or 1 tablespoon dried rosemary and steep for 15 minutes. Strain and pour over your hair after a shampoo and clear water rinse. Do not rinse again.

Dandruff

The stinging nettle rinse is best for a mild case. For a persistently itchy and/or flaky scalp, dry hair, or split ends, try the oil massage and herb rinse.

Stinging Nettle Rinse. Combine 3 heaping tablespoons of stinging nettle with 2 cups boiling water and simmer for 20 minutes. Cool to a comfortable temperature and strain. Use as a rinse after washing and rinsing the hair. Do not rinse off.

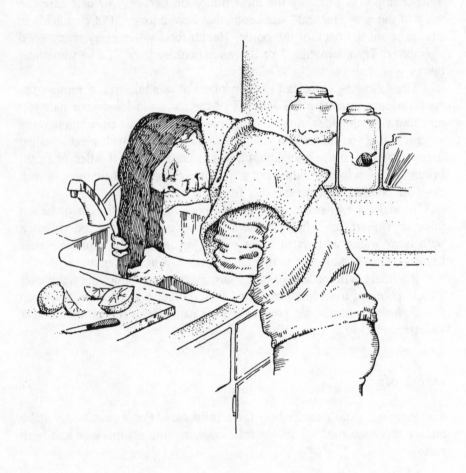

Oil Massage and Herb Rinse. Massage 1/2 to 1 teaspoon wheat germ or olive oil into your scalp 1 hour before shampooing. Then prepare the rinse by bringing 2 quarts water to a boil. Add 1/2 cup nettle leaves and 1/4 cup comfrey leaves and simmer for 10 minutes. Strain and add 1/4 cup apple cider vinegar. Let cool and use 1 quart as a rinse. Refrigerate the second quart and massage some into the scalp each day or whenever any itching or flakiness returns.

Vitamin A. Vitamin A is essential for healthy skin. Take a daily supplement of 10,000 I.U. or 1 cup of carrot juice daily until the condition clears.

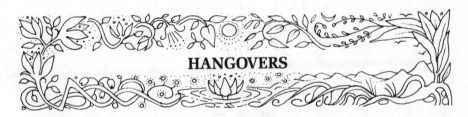

HANGOVERS

Of course, the best prevention is to abstain from alcohol or at least be moderate in your consumption. I've noticed that many people who over-indulge in alcohol are extremely sensitive people who use alcohol in order to numb themselves so they won't feel their pain and their difference, so that they'll be more like other people.

Rose quartz is a beautiful pink stone that will help you to love and nurture yourself, and to believe that you are worthy of love. It helps you to heal the child within. If you carry with you a piece about the diameter of a quarter, it will help to alleviate the need to drink.

But if you do tend to overindulge, before you go out drinking, or at least before you go to bed that night, take extra vitamins B and C and calcium and drink plenty of fluids, not including alcohol or coffee, which are both diuretics.

If you do get a hangover, the following remedies may be helpful.

Tomato Juice. Drink 1 glass, slowly. This is a time-honored remedy.

Acupressure Massage. The next morning it helps to rub acupuncture point S45, located on the second toe just above the upper corner of the nail on the third toe side. (S is for stomach.) Rub this area firmly with a circular motion, using your thumb, for 2 to 3 minutes (no longer).

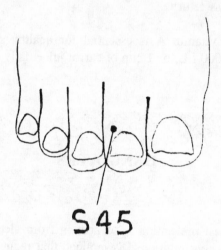

S45

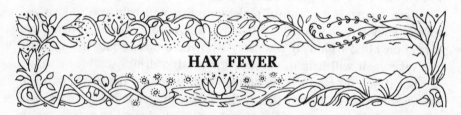

HAY FEVER

Hay fever is caused by sensitivity to airborne pollens and mold spores. Spring, when the air is heavy with pollens from grasses and trees, is often a prime time for hay fever reactions. East of the Rocky Mountains, the peak of the regional hay fever season occurs between mid-August and mid-September, when the ragweed plant is producing the most pollen. In the Midwest, attacks of hay fever are common when mold spores are released as the wheat, barley, and corn ripen.

Hay fever is characterized by sneezing, itchy and watery eyes, running nose, and burning throat and palate. It can lead to lack of sleep; loss of appetite; inflammation of the ears, sinuses, throat, and bronchi, as well as asthma. And it can lower the body's resistance to other diseases.

Hay fever tends to occur among people who are overly sensitive to their environment. Sometimes these people were overprotected as children, and they do not feel that the world is a safe place for them.

Vitamin A. Massive amounts of this vitamin have been used *preventatively* with excellent results. But it must be emphasized that it will not work after the symptoms have begun. This treatment should start 4 months *before* the expected hay fever season begins, and then continue throughout the season.

For best results, also take vitamin E to prevent vitamin A from being destroyed by oxygen, and lecithin to increase the absorption of vitamin A. Your daily regimen should be: 50,000 I.U. vitamin A, 200 I.U. vitamin E, and 2 capsules lecithin.

Note: Some people are concerned about the possible toxicity of taking too much vitamin A. According to Adele Davis, toxicity has only been observed in people taking over 100,000 units per day *for over a year.* Vitamin A therapy is *not* recommended for pregnant women.

Vitamin C. Vitamin C is a natural antihistamine that also detoxifies foreign substances entering the body. Histamines are normal body chemicals that are believed to cause the symptoms of hay fever and other allergies. Antihistamines are commonly used to relieve—though not cure—the symptoms of hay fever. Common side effects of chemical antihistamines such as ephedrine include drowsiness, dizziness, muscular weakness, dryness of mouth and throat, and insomnia. These drugs are toxic and can harm the liver. Vitamin C does not cause these side effects.

The best way to use vitamin C is preventatively. For example, take 1000 mg. every 2 hours for a day before going to the country during hay fever season. If you are already suffering from the symptoms of hay fever, take 2000 or even 3000 mg. per hour until your symptoms subside, and then take 1000 mg. 3 times a day as a maintenance dosage. (See chapter 5 for precautions concerning large doses of vitamin C.)

Bee Cappings. This provides natural immunity to the plants in your area. The bee cappings are the part of the wax that cover the honeycomb and usually come mixed with honey—so it tastes wonderful. The cappings close off each section of the honeycomb, so bee-keepers have to shave off these cappings in order to get the honey out. Bee-keepers have no special use for the cappings and will usually sell them at a low price.

But you must find cappings from a honeycomb within 25 miles of where you live (or where you are visiting) to get immunity to the local pollens. Or try honeycomb or even local raw honey.

Chew 1/2 teaspoon of the waxy cappings or honeycomb until it dissolves, twice a day. If you are using honey, take 1 teaspoon twice a day, plain or mixed in food or liquid.

Bioforce Pollinosan. This is a wonderful homeopathic remedy for the symptoms of hay fever, including sneezing, itching eyes and throat, and headache behind the eyes. It comes in tablet form and can be purchased at some health food and herb stores. It contains homeopathic amounts of Galphimia glauca, Aralia racemosa, Larrea mexicana, Okoubaka aubrevillei, Ammi visnaga, Cardiospermum, and Luffa perculata. It is distributed by Bioforce of America Ltd. (see Resources).

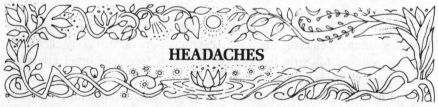

HEADACHES

Most headaches occur when the blood vessels around the brain expand (dilate) or when there is tension in the scalp or neck. Drugs are generally used either to constrict the blood vessels or to relax the muscles. Some people get a headache from not drinking their usual morning cup of coffee. This is because coffee is a natural blood vessel constrictor.

The most common causes of headaches are overeating; eating poor combinations of foods at the same meal (such as fruits and vegetables), which cause gas and pressure to the head; eating too much sugar; constipation; hypoglycemia; not crying, holding back strong feelings, trying to stay in control; tension; allergies and sinus problems; eyestrain; glaucoma;

medications; and exposure to pollution.

The following are the most popular natural cures for headaches. Try one, and then lie down in a dark, quiet room and breathe deeply. If possible, go to sleep.

Catnip, Scullcap, and Valerian. Valerian is an excellent muscle relaxer. Catnip and skullcap are good for nerves. Catnip alone is often effective for tension headaches. A tea of the 3 herbs together is also good for nervous tension.

Recipe: Catnip, Scullcap, and Valerian Tea. Bring 2 cups of water to a boil. Remove from the heat and add 1 teaspoon of each herb. Brew for 20 minutes. Reheat if desired, but do not boil.

Acupressure Massage. This works for almost every frontal headache. Begin by gently and then firmly rubbing the neck and shoulders. When they feel fairly loose, place your thumb and third finger of one hand on the 2 points, as illustrated, at the base of the skull. In acupressure, this is GB20. Put your other hand on the person's forehead. Begin to slowly and gently rub in a circular motion at the points at the base of the skull. Then build up to firm pressure, but never to the point of causing pain. Do this for 3 minutes, then ease off gradually.

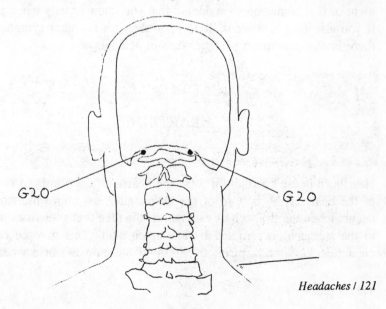

Peppermint Oil. Many people rub peppermint oil into their temples and experience a remarkable easing of tension. Peppermint oil is available in most drugstores. Some people like to use Essential Balm (see Index), which contains peppermint oil. Some people like to drink peppermint tea, or combine it with catnip, scullcap, and/or valerian. Peppermint as a tea is good for settling the stomach, and that may be the cause of the headache.

Calcium. Calcium is good for pain and calcium pills taken alone help to quiet the nerves, as well as ease pain. You may need up to 10 grams. For a more stimulating effect, take 100 mg. of vitamin C with the calcium.

When to Call a Medical Worker

If there is also a fever and the neck is so stiff that the chin can't touch the chest, there is the possibility of meningitis. If the headaches get worse and more frequent, are worse in the morning (unless you are breaking a coffee habit), or are worse at the top or back of the head, there is the possibility of high blood pressure. Other symptoms to take seriously: if there has been a head injury, or if the headaches lasts for more than a few days, or if the headaches occur more than 3 times a week, or if the pain wakes you at night or if it comes on so suddenly that you know exactly when it started, if you also have a fever of 103° or more with no other symptoms, or if there is also confusion (except after an accident).

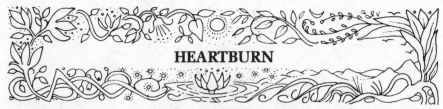

HEARTBURN

Heartburn doesn't actually involve the heart—it just occurs in the vicinity of the heart at the bottom of the esophagus, just above the stomach. It occurs when the stomach or esophagus (the tube that goes from the mouth to the stomach) is irritated by too much acid. This may be caused by cigarettes, caffeine, aspirin, or stress. If the pain is worse when you lie down, the problem is likely to be the back flow of acid from the stomach to the esophagus. If this is the case, then Dr. Donald M. Vickery suggests that you avoid eating or drinking for 2 hours before going to bed, avoid reclining after eating, and avoid tight-fitting clothing, which squeeze the stomach or esophagus out of its normal position. Avoid alcohol, chocolate, caffeine, and fried, fatty, or spicy foods. These substances are harmful because they stimulate the stomach to produce more acid, and some of them (including cigarettes) lower sphincter pressure at the junction of the stomach and the esophagus, which allows the stomach acid to move upward. Finally, be conscious of how you combine foods (see the section on Gas).

Sodium bicarbonate (baking soda) is often used for heartburn, alone or in commercial products, such as Alka- Seltzer® or Tums® . These should not be used on a regular basis because they get absorbed through the walls of the stomach, and in large doses, they can upset the acid-base balance in the body. The relief these commercial preparations provide is often short, because they may stimulate the stomach to secrete more acid. In particular, they should not be used in pregnancy because they lower the absorption of iron from the intestinal tract.

Drinking a glass of ice water may be helpful. If not, try slippery elm tea, which coats the lining of the stomach and esophagus. It also has a laxative effect.

Recipe: Slippery Elm Tea. Simmer 1 teaspoon powdered or granulated slippery elm bark in 2 cups water for 20 minutes. Strain and sweeten as desired. Drink as needed.

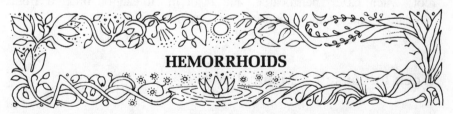

HEMORRHOIDS

The rectum is the bottom 6 to 8 inches of the large intestines, and the anus is the last inch of the rectum. The rectum is lined with a mucous membrane and blood vessels flow just under this membrane, forming a network of veins around the anus. Hemorrhoids are varicose veins occurring around the anus, and they cause pain, itching, or discomfort in the anal area. You may also notice blood on the stools, or on the toilet paper after wiping. (If the blood is actually mixed with the stools, contact a medical worker at once, since this may indicate bleeding ulcers or cancer of the bowels.) Hemorrhoids may occur inside the rectum, or they may also protrude outside the anus.

Louise Hay associates hemorrhoids with anger about past events and an inability to let go.

Fatigue and tension make it difficult for the anal sphincter to relax, which can cause hemorrhoids. Straining to evacuate small, hard feces is a major cause of hemorrhoids, because it makes the veins fill with blood.

Pregnancy predisposes a woman to develop hemorrhoids. During pregnancy, the high level of progesterone in the body causes the smooth muscles to relax, and when these relax it can cause bulging of the blood vessels. Also constipation and the natural enlargement of the uterus during pregnancy causes the veins to swell.

If there is any sign of constipation, you should modify your diet to loosen the bowels (see the section on Constipation). Also, if possible, squat during a bowel movement to enable you to use gravity and the abdominal muscles; modern toilets put the strain on the walls of the intestines.

Cleanliness after each bowel movement is extremely important in treating hemorrhoids. Clean the anal canal by dipping a cotton swab in water and inserting it to the depth of the cotton into the anus (bearing down makes it easier to insert). Repeat this action, using fresh cotton swabs, until it comes out clean. Then apply one of the following with a cotton swab: witch hazel, lemon juice (there may be some stinging with these two, but this is the result of the shrinking of the hemorrhoids), vitamin E, or Hylands Pile Ointment. This excellent ointment is made from horse chestnut, stone-root, witch hazel, benzocaine, and resorcin. It can be ordered from Standard Homeopathic Company (see Resources).

When to Consult a Medical Worker

If there is more than slight bleeding, be sure to consult your doctor. Bleeding ulcers and cancer of the bowel are extremely serious and should be diagnosed immediately.

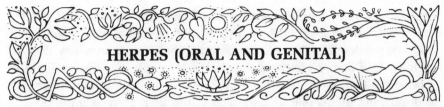

HERPES (ORAL AND GENITAL)

Herpes is a virus. It has been around for a long time, in the form of cold sores or fever blisters (Herpes labialis). A relatively new virus, Herpes genitalis is a painful, generally incurable, recurrent venereal disease (it is sexually transmitted).

The sores of herpes usually occur as clusters of tiny, red, painful blisters or bumps. They often weep and scab and have a dry ring around a moist center. Cold sores or fever blisters usually erupt around the lower lips or nose or outer edge of the mouth. Canker sores are similar, but they tend to erupt inside the cheeks or around the tongue. The external treatments at the end of this section are beneficial for both kinds of herpes sores, as well as for canker sores.

Herpes usually occur during or after a fever, following exposure to the sun, around menstruation, or at other stressful times. They generally go away by themselves within 7 to 19 days.

Genital herpes appear below the waist, usually in the pubic or anal area, or the thighs. In women, the sores may occur on the outer vaginal lips, the inner lips, the vaginal canal, or the cervix. In men, they usually appear toward the tip of the shaft of the penis. Circumcised men seem more susceptible to infection than uncircumcised men.

Genital herpes are difficult to detect in women because they cannot be seen or felt without a thorough examination when they are on the cervix, and they are often misdiagnosed when they are on the external genitals.

Warning: If you have a first outbreak of genital sores, don't assume they are herpes. Get a culture taken. It could be syphilis. An accurate diagnosis can be made by an examination under a microscope of a smear taken from the base of the sore and/or from the cervix. It should be taken while there is fluid in the blisters in order to get a proper culture. A syphilitic sore is usually single, fairly painless, deeper, lasts longer, and does not recur. Syphilitic sores are much more common in men than women, and especially homosexual men.

The herpes virus can live almost indefinitely inside the human body. The blisters appear suddenly and usually at times of stress. Typically, the blisters rupture by themselves after 1 or 2 days and leave small ulcerated areas that heal in another 4 or 5 days. Within 4 days to a month, they disappear suddenly. Then a new outbreak may occur in a few days or months. One doctor observed that for most people recurrences build to a peak and then taper off after 5 or 10 years. Sometimes the blisters fill with pus, but this is due to a secondary infection, such as impetigo.

Although Herpes labialis usually occurs above the waist, and Herpes genitalis usually occurs below the waist, there is some crossover, probably due to oral-genital sex. It's possible to verify the strain by having a culture taken of the active sores.

The first time you get herpes is the most potent. It is a primary viral infection, often accompanied by a fever and swollen glands, which can last for 2 weeks. You may feel extremely weak and sick from it. There may be considerable ulceration and swelling of the genitals, and some women experience pain on urination. When this stage passes, your blood will contain herpetic antibodies, and subsequent attacks will be much milder. This primary infection is milder with women than men, and often doesn't occur at all.

Generally, the disease is spread when the sores are present. Yet there have been reports of people contracting herpes from partners who did not *seem* to have active sores. To be fair, a person who has had herpes should always inform probable sex partners of that fact. Using a condom is helpful only if it covers all the sores.

The Emotional Aspect of Herpes

Every disease has emotional components. Since herpes is sexually trans-mitted, it is particularly rich ground for this. Most people who have herpes experience a lot of conflict about their sexuality. It occurs most often among people who feel guilty about sex, or feel conflict between their spirituality and their sexuality. Many individuals who feel that they "ought to" abstain from sex, but don't, have contracted this disease. Unlike other venereal diseases, herpes is more common among the middle and upper classes.

Before you can respond well to treatment, it's very important to work through these conflicts. Your sexual organs are a part of your being, and you need to be able to accept and love them (or, on the other hand, make a firm commitment to celibacy) before you can hope to help them. Guilt is all too often associated with sex. Yet no distinction is made between "good" and "bad" sex. Even the 10 commandments don't speak against sex; they just forbid adultery. When sex is an expression of love, which does no harm to anyone else, how can this be bad?

If you are having trouble with herpes, and if you feel in conflict about sex, find someone to talk to about it. The most important thing is to find someone you trust, and whom you regard as sexually healthy—someone you think has a healthy attitude toward sex and has successfully integrated his or her sexuality with the rest of his or her life.

If you are in a relationship that feels unhealthy, then the herpes may be the catalyst to make you face up to that. If you are taking advantage of your partner, or if you are being deceitful, or if someone else is suffering because of your relationship, or if you are having sex with people you neither love nor respect, then it's time to take a close look at yourself. You may be better off having no sex than having the kind of sex that brings unhappiness and ill health.

This kind of soul-searching will not necessarily cure your herpes (though it might), but it will help to ease the stress that brings on the recurrent attacks, and it will create a better disposition in your body for receptivity to whatever treatments you try.

Pregnancy and Herpes

If a pregnant woman contracts herpes for the first time during the last 3 months of her pregnancy, the baby may get herpes while in the womb (this is rare), or during its passage through the birth canal. A primary infection is the most potent kind, because it indicates that she had no antibodies against herpes, and so she was unable to transfer any to the child. This is the most common cause of complications with babies, and so it is strongly advised that pregnant women not take on new sexual partners during their last trimester.

According to one source, if a pregnant woman has an outbreak of blisters during the last 2 weeks before delivery, there's a 20 percent chance that the baby may get infected. If the sores are active at the time of delivery, there's a 40 percent chance of infection, unless the baby is delivered by a cesarean. Nevertheless, in the procedure developed at Stanford University Medical School, a vaginal delivery may be considered if 8 or more days have lapsed since the onset of a herpes lesion. If a cesarean section is necessary, it is performed before the woman goes into labor, because after the waters break, the baby is more likely to be exposed to the virus. Babies delivered vaginally or by cesarean after the waters break should not be placed in the nursery with other newborns. They can be with their mothers or in their own isolation room. Transmission from the mother to the baby after delivery can be controlled by careful hand washing (with detergent) and avoiding contact between her sores or objects that have touched the sores and the baby's mucous membranes. The baby is allowed to go home with the mother at the normal time unless symptoms of infection are readily apparent.

Newborns may experience herpes on their skin, mouth, eyes, or as an invasion of the internal organs or the central nervous system up to 21 days after birth. It has caused brain damage or death to half the babies who have it. It is a common cause of infectious blindness in young adults.

Cervical Cancer and Herpes

Although it hasn't been proven that genital herpes *causes* cervical cancer, women who have been diagnosed as having herpes are 8 times more likely to develop cancerous cervical cells than women who have not. If the first outbreak of herpes occurred during pregnancy, women are particularly likely to develop such cells. However, only a minority of cases develops into invasive cancerous cervical cells. Nevertheless, it's advisable for women who have had genital herpes to have a pap smear taken twice a year.

If You Have Genital Herpes

If you have recently contracted this disease, you are probably upset about it. It may already be playing havoc with your sex life. It may make intercourse unpleasant (some people find that the friction of intercourse aggravates their sores), and finding new partners may be putting you into a moral tailspin. If the outbreak of herpes was triggered by stress, you've certainly got more than you can handle now that you've got herpes to deal with, too. You may even be feeling suicidal.

Begin by treating yourself for stress (see the section on Stress). Your body won't have a chance of healing itself until you get over the stress. Go to bed. You are sick. You need rest. If this is a primary infection, you may be sick for 2 weeks.

Internal Treatment for Herpes

If you hope to get rid of the virus entirely, you'll increase your chances considerably—and almost certainly reduce the severity and duration of any outbreaks you do have—by following this regimen.

Ideally, plan to fast for 3 days. For best results, combine this with drinking fresh vegetable juices (carrot juice with a little beet juice is good) and a daily coffee or herbal enema (see chapter 4 on Eliminating Toxins).

If you can't get fresh vegetable juice, then drink 3 or 4 cups of the burdock root tea per day while fasting. Burdock is an excellent blood purifier; it encourages the kidneys and other organs to eliminate toxins from the blood. It is also good for the skin.

Recipe: Burdock Root Tea. Bring 4 cups of water to a boil. Add 1 tablespoon burdock root and simmer for 20 minutes.

After your fast, continue to avoid meat, dairy products, white flour, coffee, black tea, and sugar for another 2 weeks at least.

After the 3-day fast, begin to take the stress vitamins, as described in the section on Stress. (The Rescue Remedy can be taken any time you feel the need for it, but vitamins A and E are not usually taken while fasting.) In addition, try one of the following treatments. (These treatments can be taken without fasting, but the fasting helps make your body more receptive to the treatment.)

Vitamin C. This vitamin is one of the most powerful anti-viral remedies when taken in mega-doses. Many cases of herpes have responded to this treatment. In many instances, there were no further attacks of herpes. In some cases, there were 1 or 2 minor attacks and then no more. Take 10,000 mg. of vitamin C per day for 10 days. That's best taken as 2000 mg. every 2 hours for 10 hours. It doesn't matter what kind of vitamin C you use, so you'll probably want to use the cheapest kind. (See chapter 5 for more information about vitamin C.)

Lysine. Lysine is not considered curative, but it has minimized the effects of genital herpes, though it doesn't seem effective for facial herpes.

Many people who have used this therapy experience less frequent and less severe attacks. Take 500 mg. of lysine daily when the sores are not active, and 1000 mg. daily when the sores are present. Try to avoid nuts, seeds, and chocolate.

Acidophilus. Acidophilus has helped many people get rid of herpes faster. Take 1 to 2 tablets or 1 tablespoon liquid twice a day for 2 weeks, with milk. Acidophilus is available in drugstores and health food stores. After 2 weeks, the sores should be gone. Continue taking acidophilus and B vitamins every other day, to help prevent recurrences.

External Treatment for Herpes

When the following are applied to the sores or blisters, they help to ease the pain and speed up healing. Apply frequently.

Calendula Tincture. Calendula contains many healing properties. Order the tincture from the Standard Homeopathic Company (see Resources) or make your own by picking fresh flowers (heads only), packing tightly in a glass jar, and covering with drinking alcohol—vodka works well. Shake once a day for 13 days, and then strain. For best results, most herbalists begin making tinctures at the full moon and finish just before the new moon. Before using the homemade or commercial tincture, dilute with 10 times as much water. Swab on the sores as often as desired to relieve itching. You may want to apply it with cotton after each urination (urine does cause itching).

Hot Baths. A very hot bath can be used as often as desired to clean the sores and help relieve the itching. A hair dryer can be used to dry the sores and give relief.

Golden Seal Paste. Mix powdered golden seal with a tiny bit of water to make a paste and apply directly to sores. This relieves itching and dries them up.

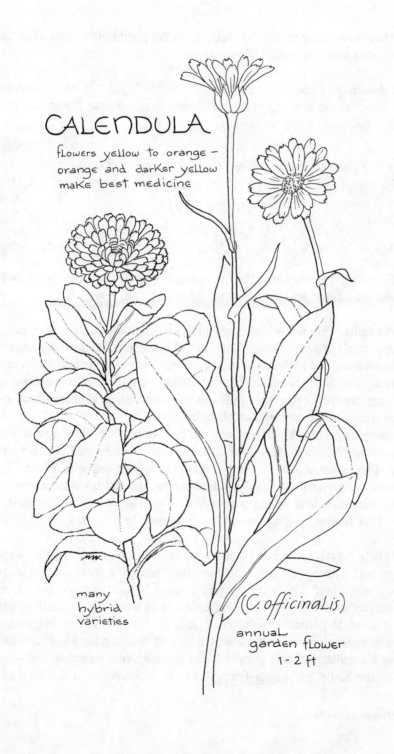

CALENDULA

flowers yellow to orange –
orange and darker yellow
make best medicine

many
hybrid
varieties

(C. officinalis)

annual
garden flower
1 - 2 ft

Aloe Vera. Apply the gel directly from the plant to the sores. (See the Index: Aloe vera for more information.)

Vitamin E. Puncture a capsule of vitamin E oil and apply directly to the sores at the first sign of an outbreak. Some people report that this prevents the sores from developing.

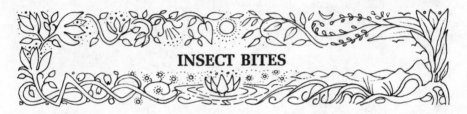

INSECT BITES

The following remedies are effective natural remedies for bites from mosquitoes, deer flies, no-see-ums, and other common bugs.

Plantain. This weed is almost universal; it grows on most unsprayed city lawns and country fields. There are 2 varieties: *Plantago lanceolate* (narrow-leaved) and *Plantago major* (broad-leaved); both are equally effective, and they give instant relief. Many people who are allergic to bites near their eyes (the eyes puff up) or to bee stings find they have no allergic reaction when they use plantain.

Macerate a small fresh leaf and apply it to the bite. The easiest way to macerate a leaf is to chew it until it is a glob of macerated plantain and saliva. This combines the drawing powers of plantain and with the healing and soothing properties of saliva. Chewing the plantain helps to release its juices, and when it is mixed with saliva, it will stick to the skin until it dries. This is usually long enough to draw out the poison.

Witch Hazel. Old Hazel must have been a really good witch. First they named a tree after her, and then they named a common drugstore remedy after her. The remedy, witch hazel, looks like alcohol. It is prepared by macerating twigs of witch hazel in water, then distilling and adding about 15 percent ethyl alcohol. It is readily available in drugstores. Dab a little witch hazel on an insect bite, and it will relieve the pain and itching immediately. It is good to carry some on a camping trip—but be sure the bottle has a tight-fitting lid to avoid evaporation and spillage.

Saliva. Licking their wounds is something animals do with good reason. Rubbing saliva into bites works well to relieve pain and itching. It's not as effective as plantain or witch hazel, but it's convenient.

Mud or Clay. Mud has great drawing powers, which accounts for its effectiveness at drawing toxins out of the body. I learned about using mud from the Apache Indians in New Mexico. They put it on their hands when blisters develop while they are working. The blisters dry and heal by morning.

Be careful to avoid manure in the mud (especially horse manure), which could cause a tetanus infection. Be sure you've have an up-to-date tetanus shot if you want to use this remedy. Clay is just as effective and there is no danger of contamination. It can be purchased at health food stores.

Bee and Wasp Stings

First remove the stinger if it is still in the skin. This can be done with your fingernails or with tweezers. Then apply one of the following to relieve pain and prevent swelling.

Plantain. Apply as directed above.

Baking Soda. Add a little water to make a paste, then dab it on. This also works well for red ant bites.

Tobacco. Moisten about 1/2 teaspoon of tobacco (from a cigarette or loose tobacco) with saliva or water, then put it on the bite. It will draw out the poison.

Mud. Apply as directed above.

Bach Rescue Remedy. Many people are afraid of bees and wasps and they go into a panic as soon as they are stung. The fear greatly intensifies the pain. This remedy helps to ease the fear, which calms the person and helps to relieve the pain. Give 4 drops under the tongue every 10 minutes until the fear subsides.

Allergic Response to Bee Stings

The allergic reaction to bee stings can result in anaphylactic shock. The early symptoms are sneezing and swelling and itching at the site of the sting. These symptoms quickly diminish and are replaced with shortness of breath, a tightening of the throat muscles, and difficulty swallowing. There is a danger that the windpipe will close off. The skin may turn blue and the person may faint. The blood pressure drops rapidly, the pulse becomes weak and thready, and convulsions or loss of consciousness may occur. It can be fatal; more people die annually of bee stings than snake bites.

It these symptoms occur, rush to the hospital. However, in my experience, the following regimen, when used immediately, will prevent a reaction. If the symptoms are already severe, follow these procedures while driving to the hospital. Hopefully, you will recover before you reach the hospital.

All of the following should be done, as soon as possible, but they are given in the order of importance.

Vitamin C. Take 2000 to 3000 mg., following by 100 mg. per hour, until all symptoms subside. Vitamin C is a natural antihistamine.

Plantain, Baking Soda, Tobacco, or Mud. First remove the stinger, then apply one of the above as directed under Bee Stings.

Calcium. Take 250 mg. every half hour or as needed to reduce the pain.

Arnica. Take 4 tablets of 6X potency each hour until the pain is relieved. This is a homeopathic pain reliever. (See chapter 1 for more information on homeopathic remedies and Resources for mail-order sources.)

Insect Repellents

Pennyroyal oil is often recommended as an insect repellent, yet most people who responded to my questionnaire were unenthusiastic about its effect. The following has been found to be more effective.

Oil of Citronella. If you can tolerate the smell of mothballs, you may appreciate this remedy. It's available in most drugstores at a reasonable price. Dab a little on various parts of your body: hair, backs of hands, ankles, and wherever the skin is exposed.

Essential Balm. This wonderful ointment from Shanghai, China, comes in a tiny 1/8-ounce vial that can be carried easily in your pocket. It is found in some stores where Chinese products are sold, and some herb and health food stores.

Essential Balm contains all natural ingredients: menthol, camphor, peppermint oil, eucalyptus oil, clove oil, cinnamon oil, white camphor oil, and hard and soft paraffin. The odor is pleasant but strong, and most bugs don't like it. The effect lasts for about an hour, then begins to fade. The balm also helps to relieve the itching when bites do occur.

Dab it on various parts of your body. It will leave a warm or hot sensation, so use it on your forehead, temples, and chin but avoid using it on other parts of your face. The fumes may irritate your eyes. I apply it with the little finger of my left hand so that I'm unlikely to put that finger in my eyes or mouth.

Tiger Balm. This can be used like Essential Balm. See the Index for more information.

Basic H. This is a soap made entirely from vegetable juices by Shaklee (look in the Yellow Pages under heath food products for your local sales representative). To use as an insect repellent, dab it on full strength. Keep it out of your eyes. Basic H also takes the sting out of bites if you apply it full strength. And you can use it as a garden insecticide to fight aphids: Just mix it with 10 parts water and spray it on.

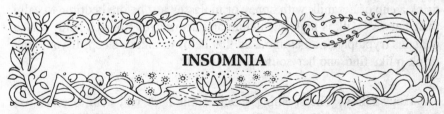

INSOMNIA

Some people need less sleep than others; this is especially true for older people. Recent research indicates that loss of sleep does no discernible harm to the body other than making you feel sleepy and irritable. The following remedies should help you sleep. But if you can't get to sleep, it is probably better to get up and do something you want to do rather than just lying in bed feeling frustrated.

Insomnia tends to occur among people who do not trust themselves, people who are afraid of surrendering to the unknown, people who always need to be in control.

Catnip, Scullcap, and Valerian. Valerian is an excellent muscle relaxer. Catnip and skullcap are good for nerves. Catnip alone is often effective for tension headaches. A tea of the 3 herbs together is also good for nervous tension. One cup of this tea will relax; 2 to 3 cups will make most people sleepy.

Recipe: Catnip, Scullcap, and Valerian Tea. Bring 2 cups of water to a boil. Remove from the heat and add 1 teaspoon of each herb. Brew for 20 minutes. Reheat if desired, but do not boil.

Sleepy-Time Tea. This pleasant-tasting herb tea is made by Celestial Seasonings and is available in most health food stores. Many people enjoy a cup or two of this tea just before bed and find that it helps them sleep better. It contains chamomile, spearmint, tilia, passion flowers, lemon grass, raspberry leaves, orange blossoms, hawthorn berries, scullcap, rosebuds, and hops.

Calcium. A lack of calcium results in insomnia. Many people like to drink a cup of hot milk with honey or molasses just before bedtime to calm their nerves. Milk is high in calcium and neutralizes stomach acid. It also contains tryptophan, an amino acid that helps to induce sleep. If you don't drink milk, find another source of calcium.

Hops Pillow. The soothing smell of this herb will help to relax you and enable you to fall asleep. Use a generous amount of dried hops and sprinkle with a little alcohol to activate the active properties of the herbs. You can make a small pillow and tuck it inside the pillowcase along with your regular pillow.

Gemstones. Various stones have proven helpful for calming people with insomnia. These include lepidolite, sodalite, and amethyst. Go to a rock shop and see which one you feel most attracted to. Hold the stone in your hand while you are trying to fall asleep, or do the crystal energization (see Index) and place one of these stones at your third eye, at the center of your forehead.

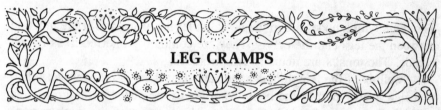

LEG CRAMPS

If you tend to get cramps in your calves, you may be feeling hamstrung about something—you may feel that you are being held back from doing what you want to do.

To stop a charley horse (a cramp in the calf), straighten your leg and flex your foot so the toes and ball of your foot are pulled up toward your knee. If you tend to get cramps in your calves periodically, the following remedies should be helpful.

Vitamin E. This is the miracle cure for leg cramps. One cause of muscle cramps is a loss of ATP, a chemical that occurs naturally in the body and which keeps muscles in a ready state of energized relaxation. Vitamin E preserves ATP, which helps prevent cramping. Relief is usually obtained by taking 200 to 600 I.U. of vitamin E daily. See chapter 5 for precautions and more information on Vitamin E.

Calcium. When your blood calcium level goes down, your muscles tend to spasm. This explains why pregnant women and elderly people often have trouble with leg cramps. Pregnant women require more calcium, and as we grow older, the hydrochloric acid in our stomachs often becomes weaker, so we are less able to assimilate calcium.

Doses range from approximately 1000 to 2000 mg. of supplementary calcium per day. Take 1 to 2 tablets of 250 mg. every 2 or 3 hours while the cramps persist. Otherwise, 1 to 3 tablets per day are usually enough to prevent their recurrence.

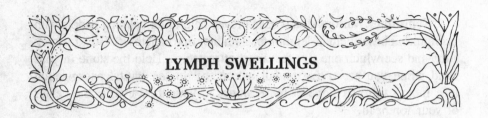

LYMPH SWELLINGS

The main lymph nodes are in the neck, under the arms, and at the junction between the legs and the pelvis. They are commonly referred to as lymph glands. The tonsils are actually lymph nodes.

Swelling of the lymph nodes indicates that there is probably an infection in a nearby part of the body. Swelling of the nodes in the groin area could indicate a genital infection or an infected sore in the thigh region, or even athlete's foot. Swelling of the nodes in the neck could be caused by an ear infection or a sore throat.

The infected nodes are usually about pea-sized when pressed gently with the fingertips. They may be tender to the touch. They may swell to the size of lima beans or bigger. In a healthy person, they should be negligible in size. But glands often remain swollen for several weeks after an infection has passed, particularly in children.

The lymph nodes are the most vital part of the body's self-defense system. If you can help them to do their work, you will be facilitating your body's natural healing process.

Since swollen lymph nodes are symptomatic of other problems in the body, these other problems should always be treated in addition to treating the swollen glands. These remedies can be used separately or in combination. For stubborn cases, use all three.

Vitamin C. This vitamin increases the number of white blood cells and enhances their bacteria-destroying ability. Begin by taking 250 mg. 3 times a day. If this is not enough, increase to 500 mg. 3 times a day. If this is not enough, try 1000 mg. 3 times a day. If there is a serious problem, such as tonsillitis, take 2000 mg. 3 times a day. (See chapter 5 for more information on vitamin C.)

Echinacea. This herb is excellent for infections because it promotes rapid healing and is also antiseptic. The easiest way to take echinacea is to buy the tincture and take 10 drops in 1/4 cup water or juice 4 times a day. Alternatively, you can take the powdered herb in 00 caps. Take 1 capsule 3 or 4 times a day. Or take the syrup as directed below.

Recipe: Echinacea Syrup. Bring 1 1/2 cups water to a boil. Add 4 tablespoons dried echinacea root (or 1/2 cup fresh root); simmer for 20 minutes. Remove from the heat. Add 1/4 cup fresh peppermint. Steep for 5 minutes. Strain and add honey to taste (about 1/4 cup). Adults should take 1 to 2 tablespoons of syrup 3 times a day until the infection subsides. The dose for infants under 3 is 1/4 teaspoon 3 times a day. Children under 10 should take 1 teaspoon 3 times a day. If this remedy causes stomach pain, discontinue.

Golden Seal. The powder made from this powerful root is an effective medicine for lymph swellings. Golden seal, like echinacea, is an antiseptic. The dosage is usually 1 to 2 00 capsules, 3 times a day. Some people will get an upset stomach from this herb. If this happens to you, either avoid the herb or else take 2 tablespoons yogurt and/or 100 mg. of vitamin C about an hour after taking the golden seal.

Green Jade. This stone has the remarkable ability to draw impurities from the body. The stone should be at least as big as the glands. Hold or tape the stones over the swollen glands for at least 10 minutes. You should feel a noticeable difference. Repeat several times a day, or as needed.

When to See a Medical Worker

If you have a painful sore throat, significant ear discomfort, a significant infection in the genital area, or if the nodes have been swollen for more than 3 weeks without getting smaller, consult a medical worker.

MENOPAUSAL PROBLEMS

Menopause is often accompanied by hot flashes, which are characterized by a sudden sensation of heat in the face and upper body and sometimes accompanied by a patchy redness of the skin. It may last up to a minute, and sweating may also occur. Afterwards, you may feel chilly. Hot flashes may recur 4 or 5 times throughout the night, disturbing your sleep and soaking your bedding.

Another symptom is a lessening of vaginal secretions and elasticity. When the estrogen levels drop, the uterine and vaginal walls thin out and become more susceptible to injury and infection. The normal acidity of the vaginal secretions changes from a pH of 4 (acid) to a pH of about 7 (neutral). The lactobacilli that thrive in an acidic environment and offer protection against vaginal infections can no longer thrive in this neutral environment. The dryness leads to irritation, and the neutral environment leads to an increased tendency to develop vaginal infections. For some women, these symptoms may last for about 2 years, and then normalize. For others, they continue long after the other symptoms of menopause have passed.

Other common complaints during menopause are insomnia, irritability, and depression. Women of nervous temperament may show increased nervousness. During this time of life, women often suffer from poor memory, nausea, constipation, vaginal infections, anemia, and edema (water retention). Many of these problems are symptoms of stress and can be prevented by following the instructions under Stress (see Index).

The usual remedy for menopausal problems is estrogen, but numerous side effects have been associated with estrogen therapy. An excellent alternative is to use vitamins that build up your body's own natural production of estrogen. The adrenal glands produce a hormone that can be converted into a form of estrogen, and the ovaries continue to produce a small amount of estrogen well past the time of menopause. Also, certain herbs contain plant substances that closely resemble female hormones, so these herbs are useful for both preventing and minimizing the symptoms of menopause.

The following remedies will help you cope with the most common symptoms of menopause. See also the appropriate section in this book on edema, excessive menstrual periods, nervousness, and insomnia.

General Remedies

Vitamin E. Take 600 to 1200 I.U. daily. Vitamin E will help to stimulate your body's production of estrogen, and it is very effective for lessening hot flashes and increasing energy and a sense of peace and well being. See chapter 5 for precautions concerning take large doses of vitamin E.

Vitamin B Complex. Vitamin B helps to stimulate your body's production of estrogen, and it is the anti-stress vitamin of choice. It is calming, and it helps to create a sense of mental and emotional well being. Use as directed under Stress (see Index).

Licorice and Sarsaparilla. Licorice root contains a substance similar to estrogen, and sarsaparilla contains a substance similar to progesterone—both female hormones. These two herbs are useful for controlling the symptoms of menopause. In England, sarsaparilla used to be a national drink, and they rarely had problems with menopause. Both these herbs are used in Dr. Christopher's Changese formula, which is available in some health food and herb stores. The formula also contains American ginseng, black cohosh, false unicorn, blessed thistle, and spikenard. These herbs are powdered and can be taken in 00 capsules; take 1 to 3 capsules 2 or 3 times a day. Alternatively, you can prepare your own tea. *Note:* Licorice is not recommended if you have high blood pressure or experience water retention.

Recipe: Licorice and Sarsaparilla Tea. Boil 3 cups of water and add 1 tablespoon of each herb. Simmer for 20 minutes. Drink 1 to 2 cups a day.

Dong Quai. This Chinese root is considered the female equivalent of ginseng. It is an excellent herb for women's reproductive organs, and it has been used traditionally by oriental women for hot flashes and other menopausal symptoms. Use as directed under Menstrual Problems (see Index).

I believe that women who use this herb regularly throughout their younger years will strengthen their female organs, causing menopause to come later in life, with minimal symptoms. For this purpose, it is good to fast for 3 days once or twice a year and drink 3 cups of dong quai tea per day for at least 3 days. (For more information on fasting, see chapter 4.)

Hot Flashes

Vitamin E or Dong Quai. Take as directed above.

Vaginal Dryness and Inelasticity

Coconut Oil, K-Y Jelly, or Vegetable Oil. These can be used as vaginal lubricants. During intercourse, the lubricant can be spread inside the labia, inside the vagina, and on the man's penis. This adds to the pleasure of both partners and makes penetration easy. Coconut oil, which is available in health food stores, is tasteless, odorless, and edible. It melts easily in contact with warm flesh. And it stays slippery. K-Y Jelly works in a similar way and is available in health food stores. Vegetable oil (such as olive oil, apricot kernel oil, or safflower oil) is also acceptable, but doesn't stay slippery for as long.

Vitamin E and Safflower Oil. Some women have found that taking 1 teaspoon of cold-pressed safflower oil and 300 I.U. of vitamin E daily helped to alleviate vaginal dryness.

Acidophilus Tablets. Insert 1 tablet into your vagina before bedtime. When the tablets dissolve during the night, the thousands of lactobacilli will help to prevent vaginal infections from occurring or recurring. This also works well to get rid of yeast infections. (See Index: Yeast infections for more information.)

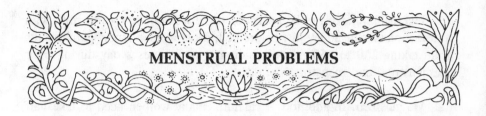

MENSTRUAL PROBLEMS

Like the moon, our wombs wax and wane. The blood circulates through our bodies, carrying hormones that influence both our menstrual cycles and our emotions. In our bodies, the days before or at the start of our period may be a time of low energy, an introverted time. Some women seize the opportunity to curl up in bed with a good book, but most women feel obligated to carry on with business as usual.

Premenstrual Tension

A few days before her period begins, a woman will usually feel some degree of tension. Many don't recognize the tension until their period actually begins. This is one reason why charting periods can be helpful. Women who lead busy lives and whose periods are regular can plan to take it easier on those days.

Studies show that 60 to 90 percent of all women have some premenstrual or menstrual distress. Significantly more suicides, crimes, and accidents occur during the 4 days preceding and the first 4 days of menstrual bleeding.

About 10 days before the period begins, a woman's blood calcium level begins to drop. Some characteristics of calcium deficiency are tension, nervousness, headaches, insomnia, mental depression, water retention, and muscle cramping. These are all the most common symptoms of premenstrual or menstrual stress.

Calcium. Whether or not you suffer from profound premenstrual stress, some extra calcium can make the days before and during your period go a lot smoother. Some women need just a little calcium and some need a lot. Some need it in combination with other nutrients (see below), and others can take it alone. You will have to experiment to find the right dosage for your body.

Just drinking extra milk works for some women. Try warm milk with a little molasses or honey just before bed. Most women report good results from taking 250 to 550 mg. of calcium 1 to 3 times a day during their premenstrual and menstrual periods.

Magnesium. In addition to calcium, many women need to take half as much magnesium as calcium to help absorb the calcium. So if you are taking 500 mg. of calcium, you will need 250 mg. of magnesium.

A good supplemental form of magnesium is the cell salt magnesia phosphorica (mag phos or phosphate of magnesium), which is available from the Standard Homeopathic Company (see Resources). It comes in tiny milk sugar tablets that dissolve in your mouth. Take 5 to 8 of these 3X potency tablets every 30 to 60 minutes, more or less, as needed.

Vitamin A. This vitamin is necessary for the absorption of calcium. If you are not getting enough of this nutrient in your diet (see chapter 5 on Vitamins and Minerals), take 10,000 I.U. with your calcium.

Vitamin D. This is another important nutrient for calcium absorption. If you aren't getting much sunlight or drinking vitamin D enriched milk, then consider taking 400 I.U. with your calcium.

Vitamin B Complex. This is the stress vitamin, and some women report relief from premenstrual stress by increasing their dietary or supplementary intake of this vitamin.

Chamomile Tea. This is soothing to the nerves. Drink 1 to 3 cups per day.

Recipe: Chamomile Tea. Cover 1 to 3 teaspoons of chamomile with 1 cup boiling water. Add peppermint or other herbs, if desired. Brew in a covered container for 5 minutes.

Water Retention (Edema)

Many women experience water retention just before their period begins.

Their breasts may swell and become tender; there may be puffiness around the wrists, fingers, ankles, under the eyes; there may be a swelling of the abdomen and a weight gain of up to several pounds.

Edema occurs when abnormal amounts of fluid pass out of the blood vessels and into the tissue spaces. This can be caused by a low protein diet. Birth control pills are another cause, as is a high premenstrual level of estrogen or a low blood calcium level. The following remedies have been effective.

Vitamin B6. B6 should always be taken as part of the B complex. Try 10 to 50 mg. a day. Experiment to find the best dosage for yourself.

Calcium. Calcium alone or in combination with magnesium can be helpful. See above.

Asparagus. Asparagus is a natural diuretic. Many women report relief within an hour of eating several stalks of fresh, frozen, or canned asparagus. However, any diuretic will wash out water-soluble vitamins, so wait until after you urinate and then take extra vitamin B complex (a natural tablet that contains 5 to 10 mg. of B2 and B6, or a tablespoon of brewer's yeast) and vitamin C (about 100 mg).

Missed Period

Possible causes of a missed period are pregnancy, traveling, severe stress, congenital defect of the genital tract, hormone imbalance, cysts or tumors, endometriosis (excessive growth of the lining of the womb), pituitary failure, underweight (being 10 to 15 percent below a healthy minimum weight can stop your periods), weak thyroid (hypothyroidism), too much estrogen, extreme iron deficiency, extreme change in diet, or a vitamin B12 deficiency (especially in strict vegetarians).

A missed period can be treated with natural remedies. Emmenagogues are herbs that will bring on a late period but will not induce an abortion if pregnancy is the cause of the missed period. Abortifacients will not necessarily bring on a late period, but they often will induce an abortion. Some herbs, like pennyroyal, combine both properties. Black cohosh is a strong emmenagogue, but is not generally recognized as an abortifacient, though some herbalists recommend against using it during the first trimester. The first remedy to consider, before herbs, is diet, a common cause of the cessation of menstrual periods.

Diet. Women on fruitarian, raw foods, mucusless, or other extreme diets often miss periods. Some advocates of these diets claim that cessation of menstrual periods is healthy; that the body is reabsorbing the menstrual fluids and ovulation is still taking place. Whether or not this is true, most women whose periods have stopped do not feel healthy and would like to begin menstruating again. This can generally be accomplished by broadening the diet to include more protein.

Black Cohosh. This herb has been praised by many women for successfully bringing on their periods. Drink 3 cups of tea a day and expect results in 1 to 3 days.

Recipe: Black Cohosh Tea. Use 1 teaspoon of black cohosh per cup of boiling water and simmer for 10 minutes.

Pennyroyal. Since this herb is both an emmenagogue and an abortifacient, it will help to bring on your period regardless of the cause of the delay. However, if you suspect you are pregnant and want to keep the baby, don't use this herb. And if you do use it, don't be surprised if your period is heavier than usual; pennyroyal will cause a heavy flow. Drink 1 to 3 cups of tea per day. Discontinue or use less if painful cramping or other discomfort occurs. *Note*: This is not intended as an abortifacient remedy.

Recipe: Pennyroyal Tea. Pour 1 cup boiling water over 1 to 2 teaspoons pennyroyal and brew in a covered container for 5 minutes.

Vitamin E. This vitamin has been used by many women who have a long history of missed periods. Its potency may be related to its importance in the functioning of the pituitary and adrenal glands. I suggest experimenting with dosages between 400 and 800 I.U. taken daily for 1 to 10 days before the next period is due. (See chapter 5 for precautions concerning taking vitamin E.)

Orgasm. An orgasm sometimes causes the flow to start, perhaps because it contracts the uterus.

Exercise. Headstands are particularly recommended by many women, perhaps because the position allows postural draining.

Irregular Periods

A certain amount of irregularity occurs naturally as a response to stress, tension, long trips, and climate. However, consistent irregularity could be a sign of pituitary or thyroid problems or tumors in the uterus or ovaries. Discontinuing birth control pills may result in irregular periods. Another cause may be moderate to heavy use of marijuana, particularly during adolescence. Women between the ages of 40 and 55 could be experiencing signs of approaching menopause.

Dong Quai. Dong quai has been used by oriental women to nourish the female glands and to regulate monthly periods for thousands of years. The easiest way to take this herb is to purchase the whole dried root and nibble off a pea-size piece once or twice a day and let it dissolve slowly in your mouth.

Vitamin E. Experiment with dosages between 400 and 800 I.U., taken daily or from 1 to 10 days before the next period is due. (See chapter 5 for precautions concerning taking vitamin E.)

Lunaception. This is a method of regulating your cycle, developed by Louise Lacey and described in her book, *Lunaception* (now out of print, but copies can be ordered from Louise Lacey at Box 489, Berkeley, CA 94701). The idea of lunaception is based on mimicking the light of the full moon, which shines brightly for three nights. I have known many women who lived in the country, with no curtains on their bedroom windows and no electric lights outside, who menstruated regularly, either with the new or full moon.

To practice lunaception, sleep in complete darkness, except during the full moon. Use heavy drapes to block out street lights. Use a 15-watt night-light plugged in near your bed or a 40-watt bulb in a closet or a dim hall light to mimic the full moon. Count the first day of your period as day one. On days fourteen, fifteen, and sixteen, sleep with the lights on. Within a few months, you should be ovulating predictably on the fourteenth or fifteenth day with a regular 29-day cycle.

Menstrual Cramps

Few women escape menstrual cramps. Stress, tension, and anxiety are the most common causes. Another common cause is lack of exercise. If this applies to you, consider taking up some form of physical exercise for *at least* 15 minutes a day and combine this with the remedies given below.

If you require painkillers and sedatives to get through your periods, you will benefit from the remedies below, but you should first consult a medical worker, especially if you have fever, nausea, irregular or very heavy bleeding, general pelvic tenderness, or abnormal cramping. The doctor can screen for some of the possible physical causes of painful periods: fibroid tumors, cervical or uterine polyps, endometrial cysts, displacement of the uterus, pelvic inflammatory disease, endometriosis, or hypothyroidism.

If you don't suffer from any of the above conditions, there are still other levels to explore. If your menstrual problems began with the onset of your period, you might ask yourself if your mother had difficult menses. If so, then there may be a hereditary weakness. For example, if you and your mother are both allergic to milk, your calcium intake will be low, and a low blood calcium level will cause menstrual problems.

If your problems started later in life, you might explore what was happening in your life at the time. Many of us are like sponges for the emotions of others. Unwittingly, we absorb their feelings and become as they are, or as they want us to be. If you find you do this, seek professional help to change these patterns. Once you do, you may find you have eliminated a lot of psychological toxins, and your menstrual periods will reflect this change.

Our monthly periods are a form of elimination. The odor, color, and quantity of this elimination is a clear indication of our health and diet. If we are in good health and our diet is appropriate, the period should be painless and easy, the flow should be light to moderate, and the odor should be negligible.

If you are a careful observer of your own body, you can prevent toxins from accumulating and this will help to maintain your health and ultimately to experience aging and menopause as a natural part of life, without pain and discomfort.

I believe that the best way to eliminate toxins is by fasting and, when necessary, with enemas. Many women have found that fasting for 1 to 3 days before their period is due helps to alleviate many of their problems. Blood-cleansing teas (see chapter 4 on Eliminating Toxins) are good to use in conjunction with fasting, as is fresh carrot juice with a little beet juice for cleansing. Other women have found that fasting 1 day a week is equally effective.

This regime is also very good for the premenstrual swelling, pain, and tenderness of the breasts and for preventing or getting rid of cysts in the breast. In the latter case (and for any serious problems, such as severe menstrual cramps), coffee enemas are most effective, combined with a day of fasting (see chapter 4). If you cannot fast, at least avoid meat and dairy products for 1 to 2 days a week, and use the coffee enema once or twice a week.

By using the following remedies, most women have successfully normalized their periods. Begin by using *all* of the remedies (except the herbs). If your next period is easier than usual, you'll know something was effective. Then you can begin by eliminating one remedy at a time. If these remedies are not completely effective, try one herb a month, until you find which one(s) are most beneficial for you.

Diet. Many women find that being overweight or eating too much makes their cramps worse. Some women have less intense cramps when they eliminate meat from their diets, others have reduced their menstrual cramps by cutting down on high-fat cheeses and dairy products.

Eliminating coffee just before and during your period may also help to alleviate cramping. This may be because coffee washes out B vitamins, which are important to the health of the reproductive organs.

Calcium. Calcium alone or in combination with magnesium can be helpful. See above.

Magnesium. Many women have treated menstrual cramps just by taking magnesium. Magnesium helps to maintain a high level of ATP, which enables muscles to function and relax properly. When ATP is deficient, muscles cramp.

When magnesium supplements are taken daily for a few weeks, cramps sometimes go away altogether, so that no further supplementation is necessary, provided the diet is high in greens, eggs, milk, and fish.

According to Ray Peat, author of *Nutrition for Women*, dolomite is not an effective form of magnesium because the magnesium oxide it contains is only about 2 percent soluble. He recommends magnesium carbonate, which comes in powder or block form. He suggests taking 1 teaspoon of the powder dissolved in water, or chewing off an olive-size piece of the block each day. If this amount causes diarrhea, then take 1/3 of the dose 3 times a day. Unfortunately, this supplement is difficult to obtain, although drugstores can order it. Another alternative is magnesium sulfate (epsom salts), which are readily available. But they taste bad and act as a laxative. Try 1 teaspoon in 1 glass of water, sipped throughout the day.

Pressure Massage. This time-honored chiropractic technique works by relaxing the nerves of the uterus; it is extremely effective.

The massage can be used to relieve pain and the results will last anywhere from 30 minutes to all day. If it is done properly, it almost always works. However, the most exciting part about this treatment is its potential to *cure* menstrual cramps. This requires dedication on the part of the woman who is having problems and her support person. In order to eliminate cramps entirely, it is very important to receive the pressure massage twice a day (preferably morning and evening) for the 3 days before the period is due, and continuing for 3 days after the period begins. Many women have reported that after following this regime for 3 months, their cramps did not return and further massage was unnecessary. (*Note:* If there are times when you cannot find a support person to massage you, then follow the instructions for Postural Drainage, described below.)

Here is the procedure. Loosen your pants or skirt and lie on your stomach. If your support person is right-handed, he should kneel by your left side. His right knee should be on the ground, and his left knee should be up so he can balance on his left foot. He should keep his back and elbows straight as he places his right palm at the base of your sacrum, so that the heel of his hand is above the little bones of the coccyx (tailbone)

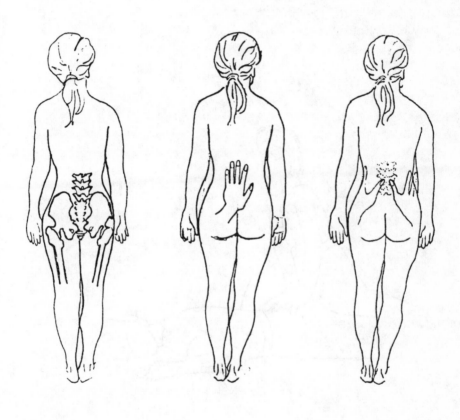

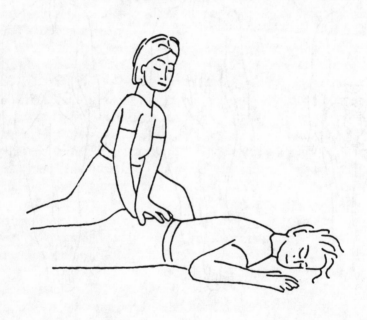

at the top of the fold of your buttocks. His head will be facing your head, and his hand will be aligned with your spine. Then he should cover his right hand with his left, both hands palm down and aligned with your spine.

Then he should slowly put his weight on his hands, gradually applying his full body weight, remembering to keep his elbows straight. He should not be afraid of hurting you, because the sacrum is design to bear the tremendous pressure of childbirth. However, if you are uncomfortable, ask the support person to let up a bit. He should hold this position for 2 minutes (which is harder than it sounds), then slowly and gradually lessen the pressure and withdraw.

While the support person is applying pressure, there may be a slight cracking or repositioning of the sacrum or the vertebrae. This is a good sign and will usually be accompanied by the sensation of letting go of tension. However, a few women have reported an increase in cramping, or a pain in their ovaries. Do not continue the pressure unless it *diminishes* the pain.

Next the support person should move his hands up to your hips, resting his fingers on your hip bones and observing where his thumbs join at the spine; this should be between your fourth and fifth lumbar vertebrae. Then he should slide his thumbs up past the fourth lumbar vertebrae to find the depression between the third and fourth vertebrae. Then he should move his thumbs outward, so that they are about 1 inch from the spine on either side. With his thumbs in this position, and with his hands in a slightly raised or arched position, he should slowly put his weight on his thumbs until you feel that it is enough pressure (this place is not as impervious as the sacrum). Again he should try to hold this pressure for 2 minutes, then release slowly. This is a more difficult position to hold because of the pressure on the thumbs.

Incidentally, this technique is excellent for any kind of lower back pain or tension, and your support person might appreciate this massage, too.

Postural Tilt. If you don't have a support person, you can use this exercise as often as you like to obtain some relief from cramping. Whenever you can't get a pressure massage during the 3 days before and during your period, you should at least do this for 5 or more minutes a day.

Get on your hands and knees and lower your shoulders to the floor, leaving your buttocks in the air. You can rest your head on your hands, keeping your shoulders as close to the floor as possible. Hold as long as you can. Then you can sag your back and straighten it occasionally.

It is important to keep the buttocks as high in the air as possible in order to obtain maximum results.

This should stop cramps. If you get cramps frequently, you should do this for 5 minutes every day for the week before your period; it may prevent the cramps entirely.

Exercise. Yoga is a favorite with many women. The cobra position, as well as shoulder stands and head stands, are also forms of postural drainage. Some women like to do knee bends, and wood chopping has also been recommended.

Heat. It's good to apply heat to the abdomen to help ease the tension. A hot water bottle that is not too full, a heating pad, or a thermophore (see Index) can be soothing.

Orgasm. There seems to be some connection between a tight cervix and certain types of menstrual cramps. Masters and Johnson noticed that during orgasm, the uterus contracts, and blood will spurt out of a menstruating woman. You can use a diaphragm to avoid the messiness of love-making during your period, or try masturbating with or without a partner. Some women have a strong need for physical contact during their periods and relief of tension may come just from having nonsexual contact with a loved one.

Vitamins. Menstrual cramps are very stressful and during stress, our bodies consume vitamins at a much faster rate than normal. To cope with stress more effectively, take vitamins A, B complex, C, and E as soon as premenstrual symptoms begin and continue until they are over. (See Index: Stress.)

Vitamin E. In addition to helping you cope better with stress, vitamin E improves the body's clotting mechanism and will help to eliminate menstrual "clots." Passing these clots is sometimes a cause of severe cramping. To eliminate menstrual clots, you will need to take anywhere from 200 to 800 I.U. a day, beginning a few days before your period is due and continuing throughout your period. (See chapter 5 for precautions concerning taking vitamin E.)

Herbs. Since one tea works for one woman and not for another, I've included five different herbs for different kinds of problems. If one doesn't help, try another.

Raspberry leaf tea is good for cramps and is also useful for easing a heavy flow.

Recipe: Raspberry Leaf Tea. Cover 1 to 3 teaspoons (depending on how strong you want it) of raspberry leaves with 1 cup of boiling water and allow it to brew for 5 minutes. Combine it with peppermint or other herbs for flavor, if you like. Drink as often and as much as you like.

Motherwort is high in calcium chloride in organic form. You can make it into a tea, as with raspberry leaf tea (above). Some women prefer to make a tincture of motherwort, which combines the virtues of the herb with the relaxing properties of apricot brandy. Motherwort tincture is also available at some health food stores. Take 1 to 2 teaspoons twice a day as needed.

Recipe: Motherwort Tincture. Put 4 ounces of motherwort in a bottle or crock and cover with 1 quart apricot brandy. Let it sit, away from the light, for 13 days, shaking the bottle once a day. Strain on the 13th day.

Pennyroyal is taken in a tea to relieve cramps. But it is not advised for women who tend to bleed a lot because it also increases the flow. One cup a day is usually enough to provide relief.

Recipe: Pennyroyal Tea. Pour 1 cup of boiling water over 1 teaspoon of pennyroyal and steep in a covered container for 5 minutes.

Blue cohosh is recommended for women who experience pain before passing clots because it is effective in relaxing the uterine os (the opening or mouth of the uterus). Women who have this problem should also take vitamin E (see above).

> **Recipe: Blue Cohosh Tea.** Pour 1 cup of boiling water over 1 teaspoon of blue cohosh and steep for 15 minutes. The taste is not very pleasant, so you may want to add 1 teaspoon of peppermint per cup, as well as some honey.

Dong Quai usually comes in whole roots and is available in wherever there is a large selection of herbs, including Chinese herb stores. Nibble off a pea-size piece of the dried root once or twice a day and allow it to dissolve slowly in your mouth. Do this for a few days before your period is due, and continue for as long as you have cramping.

Excessive Bleeding

Some women always have a heavy flow. These women may benefit from the remedies mentioned below. If you experience sudden heavy bleeding, and if this goes on for several months, or if it is accompanied by severe pain that does not respond to home remedies, or if there is bleeding between periods, then consult a medical work and have a pap smear taken when you are not bleeding. Excessive bleeding could be a sign of inflammation, polyps, tumors, hypothyroidism, or cancer.

The following remedies should diminish the flow. If they do not, take an iron supplement to replace the iron that is lost with the blood.

Shepherd's Purse Tea. This is the herb of choice for any kind of uterine bleeding. Take 1 cup a day, beginning a few days before your period is due and continuing until your period is over.

> **Recipe: Shepherd's Purse Tea.** Pour 1 cup of boiling water over 1 to 2 teaspoons of shepherd's purse and steep in a covered container for 5 minutes.

Acupressure. The point just below the center of the nose and above the center of the lips is an effective acupressure point for excessive bleeding. Press firmly at this point about 60 times a day, beginning a few days before the period begins and continuing until the flow is nearly over.

Diet. Many women who stop eating meat, or eat much less meat, experience less bleeding and shorter periods.

Alternatives to Tampons

Natural sponges are becoming popular among some women as a soft, comfortable, natural alternative to tampons. "Elephant ear" sponges are available in art supply stores and "silk" sponges can sometimes be found at cosmetic counters. Sponges with small holes are the most absorbent.

Sponges work nicely when the flow is light. With a moderate to heavy flow, it is best to combine it with a pad for protection. When you are not at home, you can carry an extra sponge (premoistened) in a plastic bag and then use that bag for your used sponge (which may then be placed in a little purse of its own to avoid embarrassment). Don't wash your sponges in public restrooms where other women may be offended.

To make a sponge tampon, cut the sponge to about the size of a regular tampon. Cut it a bit large at first, because you can always make it smaller. Before inserting, run it under warm water to moisten it and squeeze out the water. Then insert it (just stuff it in). It will bend with your shape and move with your body. It isn't necessary to use a string—you can just reach in to remove it, as with a diaphragm. But if you prefer to have a string, a piece of dental floss can be threaded through on the end.

When your cycle is over, wash the sponge in warm water and white vinegar, using about 1 part vinegar to 10 parts water. Dry it out on a windowsill or someplace where the sun will reach it, in order to kill any bacteria. Boiling will weaken a sponge, but it can be steamed in a regular vegetable steamer for 20 minutes. After a few months, the sponge should be replaced.

Diaphragms and cervical caps are also useful, but most women don't find them comfortable enough to wear throughout their period.

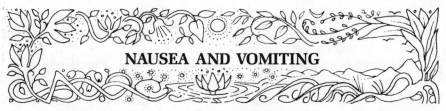

NAUSEA AND VOMITING

Nausea occurs when the nerve endings of the stomach or some other part of the body are irritated. It may also be caused by strong emotions, tension, hunger, overeating, or overindulgence in alcohol.

If the cause is emotional, crying may be the best remedy. If it's hunger, try eating something (yogurt is good). If it's from overeating, avoid food. In fact, vomiting is the body's quickest way of getting rid of unwanted material, and the best remedy for nausea may well be self-induced vomiting.

Peppermint Tea. There are many remedies for nausea, but peppermint tea is overwhelmingly recommended by almost everyone. Peppermint is a harmless herb. It is soothing to the stomach, has anti-spasmodic qualities, relieves gas, and relaxes nerves. It is also good for dizziness.

If you don't have or like peppermint, you can substitute spearmint or catnip. They are both in the mint family and are also effective.

> **Recipe: Peppermint Tea.** Make a strong brew, using 2 teaspoons of peppermint per cup of boiling water. Steep for 5 minutes. Drink 1 cup of tea and wait 15 minutes to 1 hour. If you are still nauseated, have another cup. Repeat as needed.

Vomiting

Vomiting is commonly caused by excess food or alcohol, or by stress. Vomiting is the quickest way to rid the body of what it doesn't want. Let it happen, then lie down and rest. While you are resting, consider if there is something or someone in your life that you want to get rid of. Think of how you might do that.

Don't eat anything for 1 hour. If you like, drink cool water or suck on ice chips. Then drink *small amounts* of a liquid that sounds appealing, avoiding dairy products, fats, and orange juice. One tablespoon of liquid can be sipped every 15 minutes. If this can be held down, increase the amount by 1 tablespoon every 2 doses (1 tablespoon at 15 and 30 minutes, 2 tablespoons at 45 and 60 minutes, and so on).

Wait until there has been no vomiting for 16 hours before introducing food. Then try barley or oatmeal or brown rice or something appealing, yet mild. Avoid milk. After another 12 hours, the diet can gradually return to normal.

Peppermint Tea. Prepare as directed above.

Ginger Ale. Ginger helps to settle the stomach. Ginger ale is a popular folk remedy for vomiting. Drink a small glass (about 1 cup) and wait for an hour or two. Repeat if necessary. Or try ginger tea.

Recipe: Ginger Tea. Grate or finely chop 1 teaspoon of fresh ginger or use 1/2 teaspoon ginger powder to 1 cup boiling water. Simmer for 20 minutes.

When to Call a Medical Worker

If the nausea lasts for more than a few days, or if there has been a head injury, you should contact a health care provider. In a diabetic, nausea may be an early sign of an impending diabetic coma. Nausea could be connected with a bladder infection or ulcers, gall bladder, or intestinal problems. Some medications cause nausea. If you are on a new medication, call the doctor who prescribed it.

If the vomiting lasts more than a day; or if violent retching goes on for more than 2 hours; or if fluids can't be held down for 10 to 12 hours in anyone over 10 years old, for 8 hours in a child 2 to 6 years old, or for 6 hours in a child under 2 years old; if there is blood in the vomit; or if there is severe or prolonged pain; or if abdominal pain is severe or constant and isn't relieved by the passing of gas or stools, call a medical worker.

If vomiting follows a blow to the head, this may indicate swelling of the brain or bleeding inside the skull. If there is also chest pain, a heart attack should be suspected. If there is also pain on the lower right side of the pelvic area, appendicitis should be considered. If home-canned foods or meats that have been improperly refrigerated have been consumed within the last 36 hours, suspect botulism.

Vomit that looks like coffee grounds could be a sign of bleeding in the upper alimentary tract. Vomit ejected with great force could be a sign of congenital pyloric obstruction.

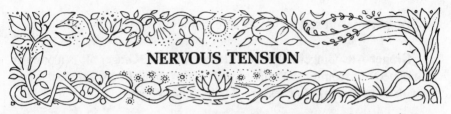

NERVOUS TENSION

It is important to get daily exercise (preferably outdoors), adequate sleep, a good diet, and some pleasure in your life. If you aren't getting these things, then don't expect miracles from any herbal remedy. If you live under conditions of constant stress, you may want to re-evaluate your lifestyle.

Nervous tension often develops as a result of personal problems. Until the cause of the tension is overcome, any remedy will be only temporary. If something is seriously bothering you, find a friend or therapist whom you can trust. When grief or anger are repressed, they come out as sickness and tension in your body.

The food you eat feeds your nerves. Refined foods (white sugar and white flour) are "empty"—the essential vitamins and minerals have been removed. Yet these foods require B vitamins for their assimilation, so they rob your body of its store of B vitamins for their own digestion. A lack of B1 causes nervous irritability, insomnia, poor memory, and vague fears. A lack of B2 causes degeneration of nervous tissues and mental confusion. A lack of B3 causes depression, irritability, fatigue headaches, vague aches and pains, and memory loss. A lack of B12 causes tiredness, poor appetite, and pain and stiffness in the spine.

Resist any temptation to take tranquilizers or alcohol; they are brain depressants and easily set up a pattern of dependency. Marijuana creates problems of dependency, grogginess, and lack of motivation. Nervous people tend to drink a lot of coffee, which gives a temporary "lift," but also taxes the nerves, leaving them more nervous than ever and badly in need of another cup of coffee. By the end of the day, it's not surprising the body finds it difficult to sleep. The coffee acts as a diuretic, washing out water-soluble vitamins, which include B and C.

Massage is a favorite remedy for tension. The healing power of touch combines with the tangible benefit of relaxing tense muscles. A good massage on a regular basis prevents your body from building up tensions that could lead eventually to chronic illness. Foot baths and foot massages are also relaxing and this is something you can do for yourself. (See Index.)

Yoga and deep breathing are praised by many people as being excellent for tension. The salutation to the sun and the plough are particularly helpful asanas. Alternate nostril breathing has a calming effect.

Blue and violet are soothing colors. Introduce these colors into your environment with flowers, towels, bedding, interior decorations, and so on. Place blue and purple stones around your house—azurite, sodalite, lapis, amethyst, fluorite. Sip on blue-charged or violet-charged water (see Index: Color healing).

The following herbs can be used safely to strengthen and feed the nerves while simultaneously easing nervous excitement, irritability, and pain. They can be used separately or in combination.

Valerian. This is a powerful sedative herb. Valerian depresses the central nervous system and sedates the higher nerve centers. It also eases pain. This is a favorite remedy for nervousness, particularly when used in combination with catnip and scullcap. Some people have a bad reaction to this herb and complain of stomachache, nausea, dizziness, headaches, and bad dreams (since it is also a psychic stimulant). Try it in small quantities to begin with. (See the recipe below. If valerian does not agree with you, substitute hops.)

Scullcap. This herb is very soothing to the nerves. It is also helpful for relieving sexual tension. (See recipe below.)

Catnip. This gentle herb from the mint family is very calming. It is sometimes used to prevent nightmares.

Recipe: Valerian, Scullcap, and Catnip Tea. Bring 2 cups water to a boil. Remove from the heat. Add 1 teaspoon of each herb and let steep for 20 minutes. Reheat if desired, but do not boil.

Hops. This herb, used in brewing beer, is good for relieving nervousness and sexual tension. Bring 2 cups water to a boil. Add 1 tablespoon hops and simmer for 10 minutes. Drink 1 cup, hot, morning and evening. This tea is fairly tasteless; you may want to combine it with peppermint or other herbs for flavor.

Calms Forte. Calms Forte is a homeopathic preparation that contains plant extracts of passion flower, chamomile, oat, hops, and biochemic phosphates of lime, iron, potash, magnesia, and sodium chloride. These biochemic phosphates (cell salts) are in a form that permits ready assimilation and diffusion into the cells of the body. Calms Forte are little tablets that are sold in some health food stores and can be mail-ordered (see Resources).

Herbal Bath. A sweet-smelling bath is a wonderful way to alleviate aches and pains, muscle cramps, tension, and even insomnia and headaches. It will soothe away every tense spot in your body, and if you remain in the bath for more than 25 minutes, you might fall asleep in the tub. To make the bath, cover 2/3 cup linden flowers and 1/2 cup rosemary with 4 cups boiling water. Steep in a covered pot for 10 minutes. Strain and add to your bath water.

Crystal Energization with Fluorite. While doing the crystal energization (see Index), place a small fluorite octahedron over each eyebrow. Fluorite is good for the nervous system, and this will help to balance out the right and left sides of your brain.

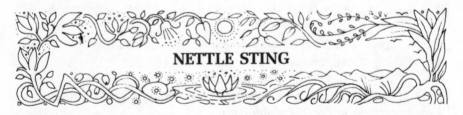

NETTLE STING

Stinging nettle is a wonderful herb, rich in minerals, and abundant in healing properties. It grows in lush profusion from spring to summer, and young plants that are under about 18 inches make delicious greens when the leaves are steamed like spinach.

Unfortunately, this fine plant has an antisocial nature; it bites. Its sting is similar to that of the red ant and can be treated the same way. But if you are careful, you needn't get stung. The tops of the leaves contain the prickly stinging hairs, but the underside of the leaves can be handled safely. Nevertheless, when you go out to gather nettle, be sure to wear leather or thick gloves and a heavy, long-sleeved shirt and long pants.

If you do get stung, here are some reliable remedies.

Dock Leaves. Learn to recognize yellow or curly dock. It almost invariably grows near nettle, and its leaves can be crushed and the juice

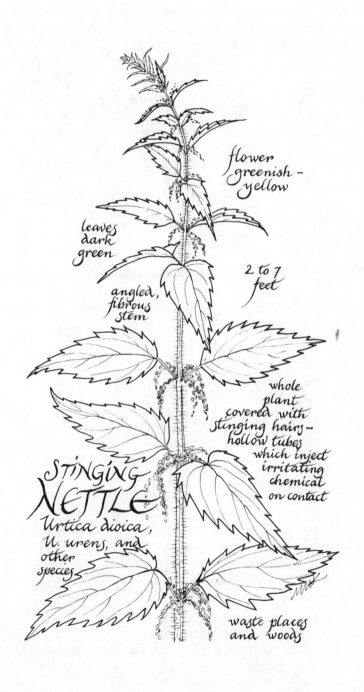

flower
greenish -
yellow

leaves
dark
green

2 to 7
feet

angled,
fibrous
stem

whole
plant
covered with
stinging hairs —
hollow tubes
which inject
irritating
chemical
on contact

STINGING
NETTLE

Urtica dioica,
U. urens, and
other
species

waste places
and woods

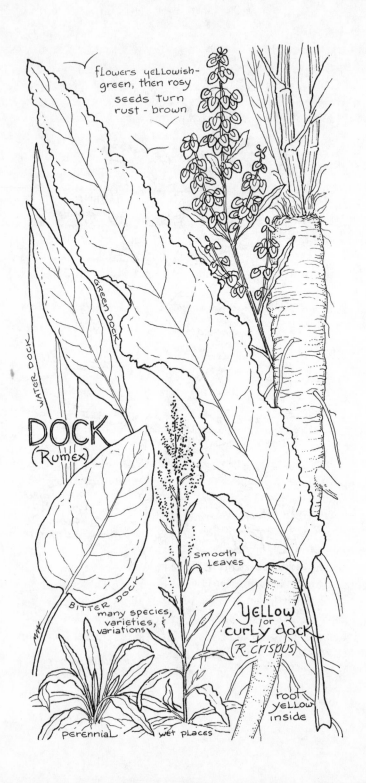

flowers yellowish-
green, then rosy
seeds turn
rust - brown

WATER DOCK

GREEN DOCK

DOCK
(Rumex)

BITTER DOCK

many species,
varieties, &
variations

smooth
Leaves

Yellow
or
curLy dock
(R. crispus)

root
yellow
inside

PERENNIAL   wet places

applied to the skin to remove the sting of the nettle. Nature, in her perfect wisdom, provides the cure for the ailments she creates.

Bracken Fern. Many people claim that the juice from the leaves of this lovely fern—which also tends to grow near nettles—can be used to relieve the sting of nettle. It does help, but I find dock much more effective.

Baking Soda. If you can't find dock or bracken, the old stand-by is a paste made from baking soda and water. Apply to the skin where it stings.

Mud or Clay. This is excellent to draw out the poison. Apply a thin layer over the skin and let it dry. Ideally, use mud from the area where the nettle grows. Be careful not to use mud that has animal manure in it, and don't use this remedy if you haven't had a tetanus shot within the last 8 years.

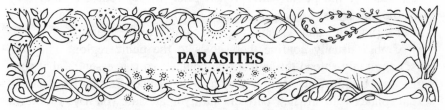

PARASITES

The parasites discussed in this section include lice, scabies, pinworms, and ticks. If you are suffering from an infestation of any kind, it is appropriate to ask yourself, "What's bugging me?" There is probably someone or something that is sucking at your life's blood.

The following general sanitary measures will help to contain an infestation, particularly of lice.

First, vacuum all rugs, floors, and furniture. Collect all clothing, bedding, and uncovered pillows. If there are children, include stuffed animals and dress-up clothes and wigs. These do not necessarily need to be washed, but they must be put in a hot dryer for at least 20 minutes, or isolated for at least 10 days, or dry-cleaned. This should be repeated just before each treatment. Change clothes daily, or at least after each bath.

Isolate each person's towel, washcloth, comb, hair brush, and personal belongings. For head lice, soak the comb and brush in a solution of 1 part bleach (or Pine-Sol® or ammonia) and 10 parts water for 15 minutes.

Clean the toilet seat after each use (not necessary for head lice). Bleach, Pine-Sol® , or ammonia are good disinfectants.

Those with head lice should avoid contact with other people's hair. Don't sleep in other people's beds or encourage them to sleep in yours. Avoid public swimming places.

The following remedies should clear up the problem. If you have tried various remedies and the parasites keep returning or flatly refuse to leave, see a homeopathic doctor. A good homeopath will spend at least half an hour talking to you about your physical, mental, emotional, and spiritual state of being, and then will select the proper remedy for you.

Pubic Lice ("Crabs")

This parasite is often found when there is a persistent itch in the pubic hairs. Careful inspection may reveal tiny white or transparent creatures on the skin at the base of the pubic hairs. When pried loose from the skin, they resemble tiny crabs. Look also for eggs (nits), which are mere specks, the size of a pinpoint, and which cling tenaciously to the hairs.

"Crabs" usually confine themselves to the pubic region. They are most commonly spread through sexual contact, so it is essential that your partner(s) be informed, and that they also be treated. Refrain from having sexual contact with any new partners until you are sure you have gotten rid of the parasite to avoid spreading the disease. Be sure to follow the general sanitary measures given at the beginning of this section.

Children rarely get pubic lice since they don't have pubic hairs, but occasionally these parasites will be found on the eyelashes or the hairline of children. See below for the treatment of lice on the eyelashes. Treat pubic lice on the hairline the same as head lice.

The following drugs are the most common and effective remedies for crabs, as well as other lice and scabies.

Pyrinate A200. This is a relatively natural drug that is sold at most drugstores, at a reasonable price, and without a prescription. The active ingredient is pyrethrum, which is a flower (*Chrysanthemum cinerariae folium*) that contains pyrethrins. Pyrethrum is rapidly toxic to many insects, acting on their nervous systems to produce muscular excitation, convulsions, and paralysis. It has a much quicker knock-down effect than benzene hexachloride (Kwell®), which is the medication most doctors prescribe, but it is less persistent and less stable. After application, comb with a fine-toothed comb to remove nits. The treatment should be repeated after 1 week. Pyrinate is usually effective, but if it doesn't work after 1 or 2 treatments, or if you don't want to take any chances because you expect to have contact with an unexposed person, you may have to use Kwell® .

Kwell® (gamma benzene hexachloride, GBH). The active ingredient in Kwell® is an extremely potent chlorinated insecticide that breaks down very slowly and meanwhile contaminates the environment. It is used externally, but if it is accidentally eaten or inhaled, it is stored in body fat. Some people are allergic to hexachlorides.

The greatest concern about Kwell® is that it can be absorbed directly through the skin. This is especially true of children, whose skin is much softer and more penetrable. The danger of Kwell® to the individual (aside from the danger to the environment) depends mostly on how much is used, how often, how large an area of the body is covered, and whether it is used by children or adults. When it is used for pubic or head lice, it is only applied to a small area of the body, and it is removed after a short period of time. But when it is used for scabies, it is applied to the whole body and must be left on for 24 hours.

Two medical journals, *The Medical Letter* and the *Journal of the American Medical Association*, have expressed concern about the misuse of Kwell® , and the use of Kwell® for children who have scabies. They caution against using too much at once, and against using it more than 1 or 2 times. Convulsions and death have occurred in animals after ingesting Kwell® or absorbing large amounts through the skin. Convulsions have been reported in children after external use, but in most cases, use was excessive or prolonged, or accidentally ingested. Both of these journals recommend sulfur in petrolatum for children with scabies, instead of Kwell® .

If Kwell® is used at all (a prescription is required), it should be used with extreme caution (follow the directions on the bottle). Where possible, dump the Kwell® -contaminated water where the environment won't be too adversely affected. I suggest taking vitamin C for detoxification: 500 mg. 4 times a day for the day before and the day of the treatment. On the next day take 250 mg. 4 times a day. And on the the fourth day, take 250 mg. twice a day. Use the same dosage for children.

Crabs on Eyelashes

When crabs are on the eyelashes, they burrow in at the edge of the eye-lids. They look like small moles, and they itch. There may be only 1 or 2. Attempts to remove these with the fingernails are generally futile, and applying Rid® or Kwell® is irritating to the eyes and ineffectual.

Needle. Crabs on the eyelashes can be easily and gently pried loose by using a needle or straight pin, and then they can be removed with tweezers. Of course, be extremely careful about using a needle near the eye, especially with small children. Reassure them that it will not be painful because the needle is only used to separate the crab from the eyelid.

Nits on the Eyelashes and Eyebrows

Vinegar. Dip a cotton swab into a bottle of full-strength vinegar and apply to the lashes or eyebrows. Then the nits will slide off if you grasp them between your fingernails.

Head Lice (Pediculosis capitis)

Adult lice are rarely seen but tiny eggs (nits) can be found clinging to the hairs, within an inch of the scalp. They look very much like dandruff, but cannot be brushed aside. They are most commonly found behind the ears and around the nape of the neck. In serious cases, the lymph glands in the neck or under the arms may swell.

Pyrinate A200, Cuprex® , or Rid® . As described above under Pyrinate A200, these remedies are usually effective for head lice when combined with nit-picking.

Nit-Picking. After treating the scalp, comb the hair with a fine-tooth comb, and then carefully and methodically inspect the head. Dead eggs slide off the hair easily, live eggs have to be grabbed between the fingernails before they will slide off. Carefully dispose of the live eggs.

Kwell® . If all else fails, Kwell® can be used as a last resort. See the discussion above.

Scabies

Scabies are caused by an infestation of mites. It takes about 1 hour for the adult female to submerge herself below the skin, so it is worthwhile to wash thoroughly and immediately if you have been exposed to someone with scabies. The submerged female remains under the skin for her full life span, which is about 30 days. A few hours after her arrival, she lays her first egg, which is about half her own length. She lays 2 or 4 eggs each day. She stays in the upper layer of the skin, creating a kind of burrow that can be seen as a short, wavy, dirty-looking line with a tiny blister at the end.

The eggs hatch in 3 or 4 days. After about 1 day, the young will move to the surface of the skin to find their own burrows. They will mature in 10 to 14 days. Most mites are found on the hands and wrists. They do not disturb the back. But immature mites may seek out thinner skin, resulting in a rash in the armpits, elbows, lower buttocks, thighs, waist, the backs of the forearms, backs of the calves, ankles, feet, penis, and scrotum. They cannot survive without a host for more than 2 weeks. Cold immobilizes them at 16° C.

Like crabs, scabies are transmitted through intimate personal contact, but they may also be transmitted through towels, bedding, or clothing. Scabies prefer children and young adults.

Itching may intensify at night, when they are warm, and when clothes are removed. Scratching may lead to secondary infections, such as staph or strep.

The standard treatment for scabies is Kwell® , but this is toxic, particularly for children whose thin skin absorbs easily. (See the description of Kwell® above.) It is applied to the whole body, except the eyes and mucous membranes and is left on for 24 hours. A second application may be necessary 1 week later. The remedies below are usually effective. Use all three remedies together.

Tincture of Green Soap. This is available in any drugstore. Begin in the evening by taking a hot bath and lathering with tincture of green soap (if available, add 25 percent strength tincture of calendula) and scrub the skin vigorously, preferably with a soft brush, to help open up the burrows. Rinse and dry.

Oil of Lavender. Apply all over the body twice a week for 2 weeks.

Sulfur 3X. This is a homeopathic remedy. Take 4 tablets 3 times a day for 2 weeks (see Resources for mail-order sources).

Pinworms

Pinworms are tiny white roundworms less than 1/2 inch long and about the thickness of a straight pin. They live in the upper part of the large intestine, near the appendix, and must travel to the outside of the anus to lay their eggs. The female comes out at night and secretes an irritating substance around the anus, into which she lays her eggs.

Pinworms can be diagnosed on sight. An adult who experiences anal itching, primarily at night, can examine himself or herself when the itching occurs by moistening a cotton swab with vegetable oil and inserting it into the anus and then withdrawing it and observing if there are any pinworms there. This may need to be done several times.

With children who cry out at night and try to scratch the anus, go into the darkened room with a flashlight and examine the anal area. Another way to diagnose pinworms is to look carefully at the feces to see if there are any little white worms there.

If you haven't actually seen a pinworm, but the itching persists and does not seem to be caused by hemorrhoids, a simple test can be performed by wrapping a piece of scotch tape around your finger, sticky side out and touching it to the anus. This should be done before getting up in the morning. If there are any eggs there, they will adhere to the tape. Then the tape should be folded in on itself (sticky sides together) and taken to a lab to be examined under a microscope. It is possible to get a false negative from this test, since worms go through phases of greater and lesser activity. To be safe, repeat the test in a few days, and then again a few days after that.

Make sure your diet is good. Avoid refined foods and sugar. Be sure to get 10,000 I.U of vitamin A a day. Some doctors say that adding more salt to the diet helps control pinworms.

Pinworms are highly contagious. The eggs are microscopic in size, and they can easily collect under the fingernails after scratching. They stay dormant but alive and infective for a considerable time in dust or air, and they aren't killed by most household disinfectants. Consequently, when one member of a household gets pinworms, all members are usually treated.

Hands should be washed after using the bathroom and before the preparation and eating of meals. Keep the nails short and clean. Separate towels should be used. Linens and pajamas should be changed every 3 days while the infection is active. The toilet seat should be cleaned with soap and water or disinfectant after each use. If you don't have time to do this, at least wipe the seat carefully with toilet paper.

Clean the bedroom floor by vacuuming or mopping every 3 days. Don't sweep because that stirs up and spreads the eggs.

Garlic. Eat 1 clove of raw garlic a day for 3 days. (See Index for various ways to take garlic). On the third day, also use some form of laxative. The garlic weakens the worms, and the laxative washes them out. Wait 1 week, and then *repeat this treatment.* This is very important in order to get rid of the larva, which will have hatched by this time. To be safe (and pinworms can be very stubborn), wait another week and repeat one more time.

Mugwort Tea. This herb is well known for its anti-worming properties. Drink 1/2 cup of tea 3 times a day for 3 days.

Recipe: Mugwort Tea. Pour 1 cup of boiling water over 1 teaspoon mugwort and steep for 5 minutes. Mugwort tastes bitter, so add 1 teaspoon of peppermint for flavor if desired.

Gentian Violet. This is a natural, old-fashioned remedy for worms. It is still available in most drugstores without a prescription. The pills may be sold as Jayne's Vermifuge. Use as directed.

Pinworms in the Vagina

These can be drawn out by sitting in a pot of hot water (a sitz bath) with 1 1/2 cups of epsom salts per gallon of water. Soak for 5 to 10 minutes twice a day for 3 days. Also apply zinc oxide (available by prescription) to the vaginal opening, the opening of the anus, and the area between.

Ticks

These are blood sucking parasites. They are small and round and they burrow into the skin with their knifelike tongues. Once they are embedded, their bodies engorge with blood, and they look like a mole on the skin. They thrive in the spring and early summer in the woods, brush, and grass. They attach themselves to animals as well as humans. Sometimes they carry viruses and other diseases, and they should be removed at once. It is important to get the whole tick out, including the head, to avoid infection.

To remove a tick, put a drop or two of heavy oil, gasoline, or turpentine on the tick and the surrounding skin about 30 minutes before you intend to remove it; this will cause it to loosen its grasp. Then with clean fingernails or tweezers, grasp the body of the tick and slowly pull it while turning counterclockwise (it is believed that they burrow in by turning themselves clockwise, like a screw). Then destroy the tick, wash the area with soap and water, and apply an antiseptic, such as apple cider vinegar, to prevent infection.

If the tick has infected the area, there will be pain, swelling, and heat in the infected part. If this occurs, use one of the remedies for infected sores (see Index).

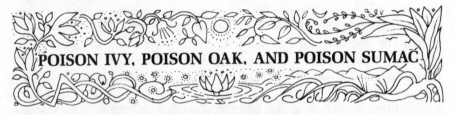

POISON IVY, POISON OAK, AND POISON SUMAC

These are all common plants of the genus Rhus (or Toxicodendron), and they all cause an allergic skin reaction. The poison is in the leaves, roots, and berries and is an oily substance. Some people have no reaction to it, whereas others develop painful rashes and blisters through direct contact with the plant. Louise Hay suggests that people who are susceptible to these poisonous plants tend to feel defenseless and open to attack. The oils can also be spread by indirect contact with clothes, garden implements, cats, dogs, and by smoke

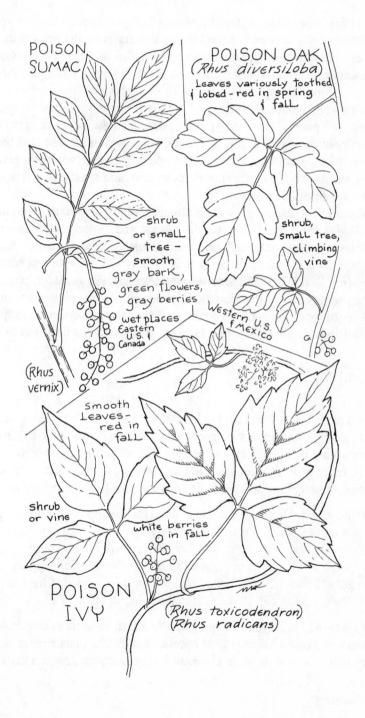

POISON
SUMAC

POISON OAK
(*Rhus diversiloba*)
Leaves variously toothed
& lobed - red in spring
& fall

shrub
or small
tree -
smooth
gray bark,
green flowers,
gray berries

wet places
Eastern
U.S. &
Canada

shrub,
small tree,
climbing
vine

Western U.S.
& Mexico

(*Rhus
vernix*)

Smooth
Leaves-
red in
fall

shrub
or vine

white berries
in fall

POISON
IVY

(*Rhus toxicodendron*)
(*Rhus radicans*)

from a fire where one of these plants is being burned.

Poison Ivy grows as a shrub or vine that trails on the ground or clings to trees and fences. It thrives along paths and roadways. The leaves grow in clusters of 3, with 1 at the end of a relatively long stalk, and the other 2 growing opposite to each other without stalks. Its greenish or yellow-white flowers bloom in June, and then the plant produces small white berries. The plant is particularly poisonous when the sap rises in the spring and early summer. A rash may occur within hours or days. The skin becomes red and itchy. Small blisters form, become larger, and eventually give off a watery substance. Then the skin becomes dry and crusty. In a few weeks, the person returns to normal.

Poison Oak usually grows as a small shrub, occasionally as a climbing vine. It also has 3 leaves, but they are lobed and look somewhat like small oak leaves. Poison oak produces small white berries. It causes the same symptoms as poison ivy, but the rash is usually milder, with less blistering.

Poison Sumac is also known as swamp sumac, poison elder, poison ash, poison dogwood, and thunderwood. It should not be confused with other kinds of sumac, which are not poisonous. It grows as a coarse woody shrub or small tree. It also has white berries. Other sumacs have red berries.

Prevention

Alkaline Soap. If the oil has been in contact with the skin for less than 6 hours, then 3 washings with strong soap, followed each time by rinsing in warm running water, may remove it. You can use yellow laundry soap (available in most grocery stores) or tincture of green soap (available in most drugstores) or kelp soap (available in some health food stores).

Poison Oak Honey. If you know that you are highly sensitive to poison oak, you can establish a natural immunity by eating 1 teaspoon per day of poison oak honey. This must be taken all year-round, though it is okay to miss up to a week or two occasionally. It tastes wonderful and can be used like regular honey. This is honey that is made by bees that have collected pollen from poison oak flowers. It is available in some health food stores.

Goat's Milk. If you can get goats to graze in an area that is heavily infested with poison oak or poison ivy, they will eat the plant without harming themselves. (Be sure to wear gloves and cover all your exposed parts when handling the animals.) The second milking after they have grazed will be the milk that you need. Drink over a pint of this milk and its effect will last all year.

Treatment

For best results, precede any of the following by washing off any possible oils, as described above. These remedies can be used for all of the Rhus plants.

Comfrey and/or Plantain Leaves. Chop equal parts of both or either one into fine pieces and then place in a mortar and grind with a pestle to release the juices. Apply to the itchy area. This draws out the poisons and prevents them from spreading. Alternately, you can use comfrey paste or salve (see Index).

White Oak Bark Soak. I've found this remedy to work when all else failed. Bring 1 quart water to a boil, add 1/2 cup white oak bark, and simmer for 20 minutes. Strain. Add the liquid to the bath. Soak in the tub for at least 20 minutes, being sure to submerge all infected parts. You should feel great relief after the first bath. Repeat the next day. The condition should be cleared within 2 or 3 days.

If the rash has just begun on a small area of your body, use 2 tablespoons of oak bark and add the liquid to a basin. Soak the affected area. If it is a very small area, just soak a gauze pad in the solution and apply to the area.

Jewelweed. Pick the fresh plant, crush it to release the juices, and apply the juice to the skin several times a day until healed. The rash should go away within a few days.

An alternate method is to pick the entire plant, break it up, put it in a pot and cover with water. Simmer until the water turns deep orange, and half the original amount of water has evaporated. Then strain, put in ice cube trays, and freeze. These jewelweed cubes can be stored in a plastic bag and brought out whenever anyone thinks they may have gotten into a poisonous plant or when they see their skin flaring up. Also the liquid can be applied directly to the skin.

Baking Powder Paste. Mix baking powder with water to form a paste and apply to the skin. This gives some relief.

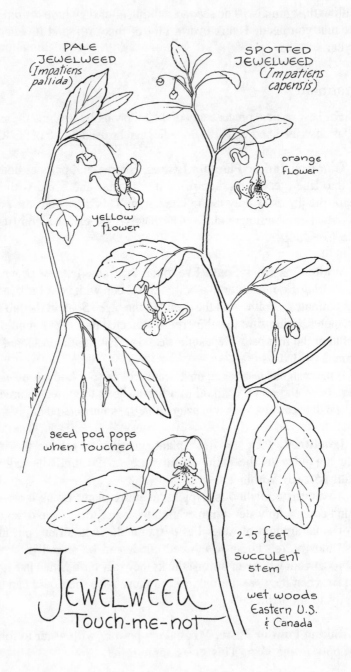

PALE
JEWELWEED
(*Impatiens
pallida*)

SPOTTED
JEWELWEED
(*Impatiens
capensis*)

orange
flower

yellow
flower

seed pod pops
when touched

2-5 feet
succulent
stem

wet woods
Eastern U.S.
& Canada

Jewelweed
Touch-me-not

Vitamin C. This is a natural antihistamine and since rhus poisoning is an allergic reaction, it helps the body to deal with the problem. For best results, take 1000 mg. every 2 to 3 hours until the inflammation subsides. (See chapter 5 concerning taking large doses of vitamin C.)

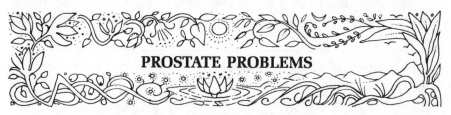

PROSTATE PROBLEMS

The prostate gland is located next to and under the bladder, and it completely surrounds the urethra. It is about the size of a walnut. There is a secretion that flows out of the prostate and into the urethra continuously, then passes out in the urine. This secretion increases greatly during sexual stimulation, and the fluid becomes part of the semen.

Prostatitis is an inflammation of the prostate which commonly occurs around the age of 30, when the minerals in the body decrease. It is usually treated with antibiotics. If not treated at all, or if it does not respond to treatment, an abscess may form, which may have to be opened and drained.

Enlargement of the prostate often occurs in men over 50. Since the prostate surrounds the urethra, it makes urination more difficult, and the bladder never feels completely emptied. Chronic constipation may also result. If untreated, the prostate can eventually obstruct the bladder completely, making urination impossible. If this occurs, the gland must be surgically removed.

When treating for prostatitis, sexual activity need not be stopped, though it is a good idea to take it in moderation. The urge to ejaculate should not be suppressed. Also, keep away from bouncing rides (motorcycles, jeeps, horses, etc.). Stimulants, such as alcohol, coffee, and ephedra tea should not be used. Alcohol is particularly harmful.

The natural treatments for prostatitis, enlarged prostate, "wet dreams," and "dripping" are all the same. For prostatitis you can also use the remedies suggested under Bladder Infections. Be sure to drink 6 ounces (3/4 cup) of cranberry juice 3 times a day.

Raw Pumpkin Seeds or Zinc. Zinc occurs naturally in the male reproductive fluid, and it is essential for normal sexual development. A slight deficiency can lead to the enlargement of the prostate gland. Pumpkin seeds are an excellent natural source of zinc. Eat 1 ounce of raw pumpkin seeds a day or take 25 to 50 mg. of zinc gluconate a day.

Saw Palmetto. Drink 1 cup of saw palmetto tea 3 times a day. If you don't like to bother with teas, you can buy saw palmetto tincture to use instead.

Recipe: Saw Palmetto Tea. Cover 1 1/2 teaspoons of saw palmetto with 1 cup boiling water. Brew for 5 minutes.

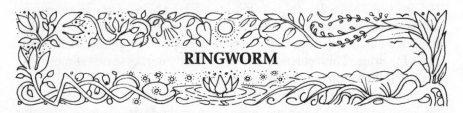

RINGWORM

Ringworm is a fungal infection that is usually found on the scalp, but it also occurs on the chest, abdomen, back, feet, under the nails, and around the groin. Ringworm of the scalp may appear gray and is hard to diagnose. It can be seen under a special light called a Wood's lamp, which causes the affected hair to become fluorescent. Infections on the rest of the body appear as reddish patches, often scaly or blistered. They sometimes become ring-shaped as the infection spreads out while its center seems to heal. There is itching and soreness. The parasites feed on dead skin and perspiration and may destroy the hair shaft, causing hair to fall out. Despite the name ringworm, it is not caused by worms, nor is it always ring-shaped.

This is a very contagious disease. Cats and other animals often spread ringworm to humans. Humans can spread it to each other by direct contact, or by contact with objects that have touched the ringworm. Be cautious about contact with other people's combs, brushes, towels, stray animals, and the backs of city buses. Even scratching yourself can spread the parasite on your own body. Wash thoroughly with soap and dry carefully because these fungi thrive in warm dampness.

If ringworm occurs in patches, just apply one of the remedies to the area 3 times a day. If it occurs under the nails or on the feet, soak the area in the recommended solution, full strength, for 1 or 2 minutes, 2 or 3 times a day.

Apple Cider Vinegar. Apply full strength.

Garlic Oil. Garlic capsules are sold in health food stores and some drugstores. Open a capsule with a pin and squeeze the oil onto the sores. Or, make your own.

Recipe: Garlic Oil. Peel and mince some fresh garlic and place in jar. Cover with olive oil. Allow to stand in a moderately warm place for 2 to 3 days. Shake twice a day. Strain through 2 layers of unbleached muslin or cheesecloth or a piece of clean white cotton.

Urine. Urine is astringent and acidic. Antibodies found in the urine can help to fight infection. The infected person should apply their own urine to the sores. This may sound strange, but it's very effective. Another technique is to mix one part urine with one part apple cider vinegar or wine.

When to Call a Medical Worker

When the lesions are extensive and do not respond to local therapy after about 2 weeks, particularly if the hair has fallen out, consult a medical worker.

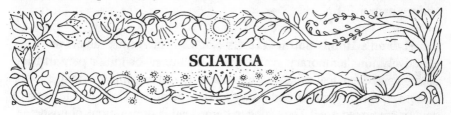

SCIATICA

Sciatica results from inflammation or injury to the sciatic nerve, which causes a pain that travels along that nerve. It's the widest nerve of the body, and one of the longest. It extends from the base of the spine to the thigh, with branches throughout the lower leg and foot.

Sciatica is often caused by tension in the lower back, which causes the muscles to tighten, squeezing on the sciatic nerve and resulting in inflammation and irritation.

Sciatica can also occur when your legs are out of alignment. A good chiropractor can re-align your back and legs, and remove tension from your sciatic nerve. This can have a remarkably beneficial effect, giving relief to a problem that may have existed for many years. Be sure to follow such a treatment with daily exercise to keep those muscles limber.

If you find yourself holding tension in your buttocks, practice tensing and releasing those muscles, one side at a time, alternately, 10 times, 3 times a day. Then if you notice yourself tightening in this area, you can consciously tighten and release the tension. In addition, take up a sport, such as running, swimming, or bicycling, which will provide you with a way of working off tension before it builds.

The pain of sciatica tends to come and go. It usually gets worse when you do a lot of standing or sitting. It's worthwhile to pay attention to your footwear; select only shoes that are very comfortable, with good arch supports. If you have to sit for long periods of time, use a good chair or cushion that gives you proper back support. Take a break at least once an hour, and walk around a bit, or at least tense and relax your buttocks.

Vitamin E. Relief is usually obtained by using 200 to 600 I.U. of vitamin E daily. Use alpha tocopherols from a natural source. Begin with 200 I.U. for 2 days. If this is not enough, increase to 400 I.U. for 2 days. If this is not effective, try 600 I.U. If no results are obtained after 2 weeks, try something else. Some people have to maintain a daily dose, and others use vitamin E only when they have sciatica. (See chapter 5 for precautions about vitamin E.)

Hyland's Homeopathic Tablets No. 22. These little tablets are used effectively for "temporary symptomatic treatment for minor pain in back of thigh and down leg; minor muscular soreness of leg; minor cramp in back of leg and foot; worse at night and in cold, damp weather. Not for severe pain or continued use." They contain homeopathic preparations of mistletoe, low cudweed, poison ivy, aconite, and wild rosemary. (When taken in homeopathic form, poison ivy works as a harmless counterirritant.) These tablets are available at some herb and health food stores, or they may be ordered from Standard Homeopathic Company (see Resources).

Acupuncture or Acupressure. Acupuncture is one of the most effective ways of treating sciatica. But if it is not available, then a good acupressure massage is also effective. The following points can be used with either method.

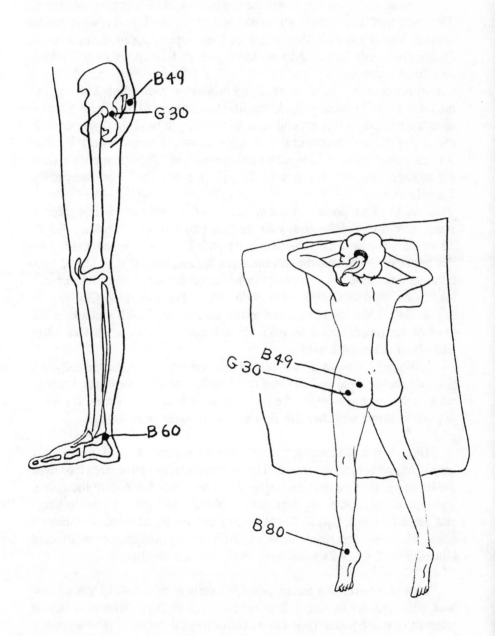

Pressure to these points should be somewhat painful, but not excruciating. The relief that follows the pain makes it well worthwhile. Pressure can be applied with the thumb, then released, then applied again, several times. Or the points can be worked with the thumb in 1 place, rotating firmly in a circular motion.

Apply pressure for no more than 3 minutes at each point. These points are most easily located by observing the illustration and then feeling for the most tender spot in that general area. No harm will be done if you massage the wrong place. This treatment should be given 3 times a week for 2 or 3 weeks, until the pain is significantly diminished. Then treat once a week for another 2 or 3 weeks, or until the pain is gone. Then treat once again, 2 weeks later.

1. G30. This point is usually very tender, whether or not there is sciatica. You can probe both your thumbs into this spot, working deeply. To locate this point, have the person lie on his or her stomach and tighten the buttocks. Look for the "dimple" or indentation at the side of each buttock. Anatomically, it is posterior to the greater trochanter. In acupuncture, it's known as Gall Bladder 30 or Huan Tiao (Jumping Circle).

2. B49. This point is located at the top center of each buttock, at the level of the fourth sacral foramen. In acupuncture, this is Bladder 49 or Chih Pien (Leaning Limb).

3. B60. This point is just behind the outer ankles. Anatomically, it's between the external malleus and the Achilles tendon, above the superior edge of the calcaneus, upon the peroneal artery. In acupuncture, it's Bladder 60 or Kun Lun (after the Kun Lun Mountains near Tibet).

Yoga. While not usually effective for curing sciatica, yoga is extremely helpful to prevent its recurrence. The asanas (exercises) that stretch or twist the lower pelvic area and the thighs are particularly beneficial: the cobra, knee and thigh stretch, leg over, locust, plough, full twist, elbow-to-knee, and the alternate leg pull. These asanas can be found in most books on yoga. They are described in detail, with good photographs, in Richard Hittleman's *Yoga 29 Day Exercise Plan* (Bantam Books).

Thermophore. The thermophore is excellent for sciatica. It is a moist heat pack that looks like a heating pad. Apply 2 or 3 times a day at intervals of 6 to 8 hours. (For a more complete description of thermophores, see Index.)

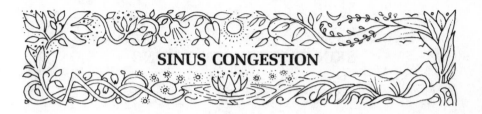

SINUS CONGESTION

If you are are troubled with congestion, you should avoid overheated or over-air-conditioned rooms (68 degrees is a good temperature during the day). Get plenty of fresh air and sleep with the heat turned down or off. If radiators or wood or oil heaters are used, place a container of water on the heater to keep moisture in the air and to keep the sinuses from getting dried out.

Sinus congestion is often brought on by an allergy, so check out your house for feathers, dust, cats, and other things that could cause an allergic reaction. You may try to remove or minimize these things for a week to see if the condition improves.

Louise Hay associates this ailment with experiencing a sense of irritation toward a person who is close to you.

Ephedra Tea. This is also known as desert tea, Mormon tea, or squaw tea. Chinese Ephedra, or ma huang, is stronger, so substitute 3/4 teaspoon for 1 teaspoon in the recipe. Drink as needed.

Recipe: Ephedra Tea. Bring 2 cups of water to a boil, add 2 teaspoons granulated ephedra, and simmer for 20 minutes. If you have ephedra twigs instead of the granulated herb, use a small handful and simmer for 20 minutes.

Fenugreek Tea. This herb is popular among naturopathic doctors for sinusitis. Drink as needed.

Tiger Balm. This is a Chinese ointment made of camphor (and sometimes other herbs) in a petroleum base. It can be found in some health food stores and places where Chinese items are sold. Apply to the area above the nose and between the eyes, to the temples, and wherever there is discomfort.

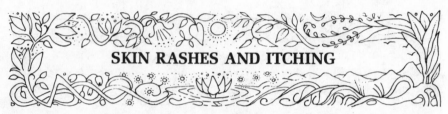

SKIN RASHES AND ITCHING

In Chinese medicine, the skin is considered one of the organs of elimination. If the related organs—the lungs and large intestines—are not functioning properly the natural outlet for toxins is closed and eruptions occur on the skin. If your organs of elimination are working effectively, and if your diet is good, then your skin probably will be healthy.

For this reason, fasting and blood cleansing are often recommended for people with chronic skin conditions. The condition often gets worse during fasting before it gets better, since the body is accustomed to using the skin as an avenue for the elimination of toxins, and this process continues even during the fast. Depending on how serious the condition is, how long you've had it, and on your tolerance for fasting, you may want to fast for 1 to 10 days. This can be accompanied by plenty of fresh juices and/or teas, and/or grapes. (See chapter 4 on Eliminating Toxins for more information on fasting and blood cleansing.)

Cleanliness is an important part of healthy skin, yet too much soap and water can be harmful. The skin secretes natural oils for lubrication. Too much soap and water can remove this protective coating, causing dry, flaky, itchy skin. Also, the body's manufacture of vitamin D occurs on the skin, when the sun's ultraviolet rays activate the cholesterol on the skin, converting it to vitamin D. Washing the skin will prevent this process from happening, so it's probably a good idea to wait about 2 hours before and after exposure to the sun before washing (particularly if you haven't been getting much sunlight or vitamin D).

If you have dry skin, don't wash with soap any more than necessary. Instead of daily showers, try daily washing of the underarms, feet, and genitals (women should avoid soap in their vagina, because most soaps are alkaline and they upset the natural acidic pH of the vagina, contributing to vaginal infections). Try to avoid creams, lotions, and heavy make-up, which clog your pores. If you are healthy within, and you take good care of your body (by getting enough exercise, fresh air, and sunlight) and watch your diet, your skin will be a radiant reflection of your good health, and you won't want to cover it or smother it.

If you avoid synthetic clothing, which prevents the circulation of air and causes sweating and bad odor, even deodorants may not be necessary. If some form of deodorant is needed, plain cornstarch absorbs odors effectively. Cornstarch can be combined with lavender and other pleasant-smelling herbs. Health food stores carry pleasant natural deodorants.

Rashes

A rash is present if the skin is red, raised, and itchy. It may be caused by an allergy to foods or to something in the environment. It can also be caused or intensified by emotional stress and fatigue.

When a rash occurs, it may be helpful to ask yourself what your body is trying to tell you. Itching often occurs as an outlet for unsatisfied desires, or as an expression of self-deprecation. What do you need that you aren't getting?

Try not to scratch, since this will only irritate the rash. You could try wrapping a towel or some coarse cloth around a pillow and then scratch at that, while having an imaginary dialogue with whomever you'd like to be scratching (including yourself).

When there is an itch, avoid wearing red or orange next to the skin. Blue is the most soothing color. Many people have cured persistent genital and anal itching just by wearing blue underpants.

The following remedies are helpful. The internal treatments are listed first, then the external.

B Complex. This is used to calm the nerves and to help cope with stress. Take a B complex tablet that contains about 10 mg. each of B2, B3, and B6, 3 times a day. Or take a tablet that contains 25 to 50 mg. once a day.

Protein. If your intake is low, get more protein in your diet, or try some protein powder.

Vitamin A. This is vital for healthy skin. Take about 10,000 I.U. a day. If you live in an area where there's not much sun, take it in combination with about 400 I.U. of vitamin D.

Blood Cleansing. This is often helpful for rashes and is described in chapter 4 on Eliminating Toxins.

Aloe Vera. The gel from this plant is remarkably soothing, and I've seen it heal a wide variety of rashes in a very short time. Just apply the fresh gel from the plant 1 to 3 times a day. Some rashes go away in a day, and some take about a month. (See the Index for more information on aloe.)

Vitamin E. You can use vitamin E cream or liquid, or open a capsule with a pin and squeeze the oil onto the rash, several times a day. It usually works within a few days. If it increases the itching, use one of the other remedies.

Cornstarch. You can buy a large box of cornstarch for a reasonable price at any grocery store, and it's one of the most effective remedies for raw or itchy rashes. Just dust it on the irritated area. If the rash is in a moist part of the body, the cornstarch may eventually cake. Just wash it off as often as necessary, dry the area, and dust on a fresh coat.

Itching of the External Genitals

This refers to any non-specific itching that is not caused by parasites or infection or a venereal disease. It applies to the major and minor lips of the vulva in a woman, to the penis and scrotum in a man, and also to heat rashes in the genital area and between the legs. Make sure there are no sores. If there are, see a medical worker.

Cleanliness is essential. Wash every day and after intercourse. Women should not use soap in the vagina, which disturbs the pH balance. Women should spread the lips of the vagina to wash in all the folds. After each urination, wipe with toilet paper that has been dipped in cool water.

Make sure you are not wearing clothing that would irritate the area, such as nylon underpants or tights or leotards, which keep the moisture in and the air out. Cotton is fine. Here are some simple remedies that are usually effective. If they don't work, see a medical worker.

Buttermilk or Yogurt. Apply to itchy area at least twice a day. Use a cotton swab or your fingers.

Cornstarch. Sprinkle liberally over itchy area. It's great for heat rash. It works well to keep the cornstarch in a plastic squeeze bottle.

Slippery Elm Infusion. Bring 1 cup of water to a boil, add 2 teaspoons slippery elm powder or granulated slippery elm, and simmer gently for 20 minutes. Let cool and apply to area. Repeat at least twice a day.

Itching of the Pubic Hairs

Sometimes the pubic area, like the scalp, itches. This is usually caused by dry skin and can be easily remedied. First, make sure you don't have crabs: Look very closely at the roots of the hair follicles for tiny white or transparent creatures which, when pulled away, look like tiny crabs. Inspect for eggs (nits) which are mere specks the size of a pinpoint that cling tenaciously to the hairs. If you have crabs, see the section on Parasites. If you don't have crabs, try one of these remedies.

Vitamin E. Open a capsule of vitamin E with a pin and squeeze out the oil. Apply to the area and rub well into the hair and skin.

Stinging Nettle Infusion. Bring 1 cup water to a boil and add 2 heaping tablespoons of stinging nettle. Simmer for 20 minutes, let cool, and strain. Splash onto the area. Repeat as needed.

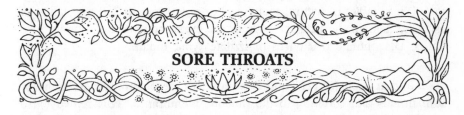

SORE THROATS

Most sore throats are viral, and like colds, they go away on their own. A sore throat tends to develop when there is a fear of speaking the truth. It is a common ailment among spiritual people who fear that they will be rejected if they speak openly about their beliefs. Viral infections cause your white blood cell count to drop. The white blood cells are the major combatants in fighting off disease, so this leaves you more vulnerable to other infections, such as strep.

If your throat remains sore for more than 3 days, or if—by looking at your throat with a flashlight—it is *very* red, particularly if there are white spots on it, or if there's a fever of 102° or more, and if the glands in the neck are swollen, you may have strep throat. The test for strep is a simple throat culture, taken with a long cotton swab. It only takes a minute, and if your doctor or local clinic is cooperative, you should be able to come in just for a throat culture—which a nurse or any medical worker can easily take—and just pay a few dollars and avoid an expensive visit with the doctor. The culture is then sent to a laboratory, and results take about 24 to 48 hours to receive—so don't wait until you are dying before you go in for a culture.

Home remedies will help speed recovery of viral sore throats, relieve your symptoms, and they will help prevent a viral sore throat from becoming a strep throat infection.

Warm Salt Water Gargle. A salt solution prevents strep by pulling the moisture out of the strep bacteria, which causes dehydration of the cells and breaks down their cell walls. The salt solution is also astringent, which means that it shrinks down the swollen, inflamed tissues of the throat. Most doctors recommend this simple remedy. Add 1/4 teaspoon salt to 1/4 cup warm water. Gargle 3 to 10 times every 2 or 3 hours.

Vitamin C as a Throat Lozenge. Vitamin C is also a powerful astringent, and it increases your white blood cell count. Hold a 250 mg. to 500 mg. tablet of natural vitamin C or a 100 mg. to 250 mg. tablet of ascorbic acid in the back of your throat every hour or two, for up to 6 hours. Discontinue if it burns or irritates your mouth.

Golden Seal, Myrrh, and Cayenne. All these herbs are excellent for sore throats and soothing to the mucous membranes. This remedy also works well for enlarged tonsils and mouth sores.

Golden seal—like garlic—is reputed to have antibiotic properties and may destroy beneficial intestinal bacteria. For this reason, I suggest using 100 mg. vitamin C for detoxification, and taking 2 to 3 tablespoons of plain yogurt, 1 or 2 hours after taking golden seal, and 3 times a day for 3 days after finishing the treatment with golden seal. This helps to restore the beneficial intestinal bacteria.

Recipe: Golden Seal, Myrrh, and Cayenne Remedy. Combine 4 parts golden seal, 1 part myrrh, and 1 part cayenne powder. Mix the powders. The most effective way to take this remedy is by allowing it to come in direct contact with your throat. Ideally, put 1/4 teaspoon of the mixed powders on a butter knife and place on the back of your tongue. (There aren't many taste buds on the back of your tongue, so this helps to avoid the hot and bitter taste of this remedy.) Swallow it down quickly with warm water. Alternatively, take the mixed powders in a 00 capsule (which holds 1/4 teaspoon). Repeat 3 or 4 times a day, as needed. (If you don't have myrrh, just omit it.)

Oil of Bitter Orange. This oil comes from bitter oranges, grown in Africa. It's effective for sore throats, including very stubborn ones. Use a cotton swab to thoroughly coat the back of your throat with the oil. You may want to use a mirror. Repeat 3 times a day, until all your symptoms are gone, and then for another day or two.

Oil of bitter orange can be purchased at herb stores and some health food stores.

Blackberry Root Tea. The root (and green berries) of the blackberry plant is another powerful astringent, and it's one of my favorite remedies for sore throats.

Recipe: Blackberry Root Tea. Bring 3 cups water to a boil and add 1 tablespoon blackberry root and/or green berries. Simmer for 20 minutes, then remove from the heat and add 1 tablespoon peppermint. Cover and brew for 5 minutes. Drink as much as you like.

Strep Throat

Strep throat tends to develop when there is a repressed need to scream. Rheumatic fever is a very serious disease that can develop as a complication of strep. This is one reason why antibiotics are always used by medical people for strep, and why patients are urged to continue taking antibiotics for about 10 days. When taking antibiotics, which are somewhat toxic, it's a good idea to take 100 mg. of vitamin C 3 times a day to counteract the toxicity. After you've finished taking the antibiotics, then eat several table-spoons of plain, unstabilized yogurt daily for several days to restore your normal intestinal bacteria. It doesn't help to eat the yogurt while you are taking the antibiotics, because they will kill off the beneficial bacteria in the yogurt. Women would do well to insert an acidophilus or yogurt tablet into their vagina each night before going to bed during and for several days after taking antibiotics.

Broad spectrum, nonspecific antibiotics are used to treat strep, which means they kill some beneficial bacteria along with the strep. This may upset the natural balance of bacteria in your body, which could result in yeast in-fections in women. Or it could lead to an overgrowth of *candida albicans* (yeast) throughout your body, resulting eventually in a craving for sweets, possible "jock itch" in men, athlete's foot or fungus infection of the nails, fatigue, depression, nervousness, digestive problems, infertility, and lowered sex drive.

There are alternatives to using antibiotics for strep. In fact, I've found that these are some of the most consistently reliable remedies. However, anyone who wishes to avoid using antibiotics for strep must be extremely conscientious in order to avoid any possibility of developing rheumatic fever. You must be sure to have a throat culture taken *after* the symptoms are gone, *to be sure than the strep organism has been eliminated.*

In addition, be sure to take at least 500 mg. of vitamin C each day for 10 days while treating strep. There were some experiments conducted by Dr. Rinehart and by the Public Health Service back in the 1930s which indicated that rheumatic fever occurred only when there was a deficiency of vitamin C. However, these reports were inconclusive, and further ex-periments were not conducted, probably because the advent of antibiotics in the 1940s detracted interest from nutritional research.

It is also advisable to take 10,000 to 20,00 I.U. of vitamin A when you have strep.

If the above precautions are observed, one of the following home remedies can be tried.

Alfalfa Tablets. This remedy almost always works within 24 to 48 hours. Adults take 10 tablets and 100 mg. vitamin C every 3 hours, until all symptoms are gone. Children 3 to 5 years take 5 tablets and 100 mg. vitamin C. Children 5 to 10 years take 7 to 8 tablets and 100 mg. of vitamin C. I've found that Shaklee alfalfa tablets, which are made from organic alfalfa, are extremely effective and are easy to swallow. They're available from Shaklee distributors, who can be found by looking in the Yellow Pages of a telephone directory, under Health Food Products. Bernard Jensen also makes a good alfalfa tablet.

"Thousand Year Old Eggs" or Preserved Duck Eggs. This remarkable remedy is made from duck eggs that have been buried for at least 6 months in bat dung, so that they are penetrated by spores which are reputed to be a natural source of penicillin. They are sometimes available in Chinese grocery stores. These eggs are almost twice the size of chicken eggs, and they have a layer of hard black substance about 1/4 inch thick surrounding the eggs.

Crack and peel the egg, being careful not to get any of the black outer substance mixed into the egg. It will be like a hard-boiled egg inside the shell. When you open the egg, the yolk will be firm and translucent black. Chop the egg and add 1 tablespoon soy sauce, 1 tablespoon vegetable oil, and a pinch of powdered ginger. Mix together and then divide the egg into 3 equal portions. Eat 1 portion with each meal. It usually takes 3 to 4 eggs to clear up the symptoms of strep. For children, divide the egg into 4 portions and take 1 with each meal. It usually takes 2 to 3 eggs to clear up the symptoms for children. For infants, just use the yolk and divide it into 3 portions and give 1 with each meal. Infants usually require 2 to 3 egg yolks.

Note: This remedy is not recommended for people who are allergic to eggs. However, one man who was allergic to penicillin tried it without bad effects.

Do not try these remedies unless you are willing to have a throat culture taken afterwards, to determine if you have definitely eliminated the strep organism—otherwise, you could be in danger of developing rheumatic fever.

Laryngitis or Hoarseness

Slippery Elm. This herb is a powerful emollient, which means that it soothes and softens the skin (in this case, the mucous membranes), reduces pain, and promotes healing. It's good for all kinds of sore throats, but it is particularly useful for hoarseness and laryngitis. Slippery elm throat lozenges and candy are available in most health food stores. Or a tea can be made from slippery elm bark.

Recipe: Slippery Elm Tea. Bring 2 cups water to a boil. Sprinkle in 1 teaspoon powdered or granulated slippery elm bark. Simmer for 20 minutes. Strain and sweeten with honey if desired. Drink 1 cup, 4 times a day, or as needed.

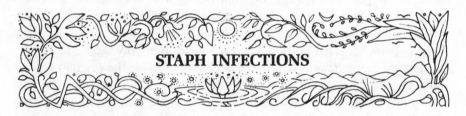

STAPH INFECTIONS

Staphylococcus is a spherical-shaped bacterium that is very common in our environment. Most of us carry staph bacteria in our noses some or all of the time. Yet it doesn't become a problem except in the presence of some combination of unsanitary conditions, inadequate diet, and crowded living conditions. Staph frequently occurs in hospitals, probably because of crowded conditions and diets that are often nutritionally deficient.

Staph infections usually occur when there's a break in the skin which then becomes infected. It is the infecting organism that causes impetigo (a skin disease common to children), boils, carbuncles, sties, and it sometimes occurs as a complication of eczema, scabies, and lice. Under a microscope, staphylococcus occurs in regular clumps resembling bunches of grapes. Diagnosis is made by a simple swab taken from the sore and examined in a lab.

Penicillin was once used for staph, but now the majority of hospital staphylococci are resistant to this antibiotic, so other antibiotics are given for 10 days. I've found that antibiotics are rarely necessary, and staph can usually be treated with plenty of patience and the remedies described below.

Staph is very common: In the United States 5 to 9 percent of the population are treated for staph infection each year. It is most common among infants and young adults.

Contagion is often one of the biggest concerns. Anyone who has any form of staph should avoid bathing and swimming in public places and should keep their sores covered while in public. This is especially true for children, who touch each other a lot. Keep separate towels, washcloth, clothing, etc.

Although staph is seen on the skin, it's also a systemic disease. It invades the bloodstream, often causing a fever and swollen glands. Therefore, it must be treated both externally and internally in order to achieve the best results.

In some cases, staph is caused by lack of refrigeration: When meat and dairy products are stored without refrigeration or left out overnight, germs get into the food, multiply rapidly, and secrete a poisonous toxin which is not destroyed by heating or cooking. Also, a protein deficiency tends to increase one's susceptibility to this bacteria, which makes it a fairly common plague among vegetarian groups that are attempting to live at subsistence level. Staph infections are also common among people who are deficient in vitamin B complex.

Another factor is cleanliness. Keeping clean can help prevent staph.

The following remedies have been used effectively for staph infections. *Note*: Golden Seal is often recommended for staph infections, but some people report that it made their sores worse. According to a lab technician in Oregon, golden seal constricts the blood vessels. With staph, you would want to bring blood to the area. The people who reported good results used golden seal immediately, with the first outbreak of small sores, and combined it with myrrh powder, which is a powerful disinfectant.

External Treatments

Hot Soaks. The most important thing is to keep the sores clean, open, and draining. People who live without running water often get infections, and it's a hardship for them to provide this kind of care, but it's essential to the healing process.

Take a hot bath or apply hot clean compresses to the area, for at least 15 minutes, 3 times a day. Add at least 1/4 cup apple cider vinegar to the bath water, or 2 tablespoons per cup to the soak water. When the condition improves, baths can be reduced to twice a day, and then once a day, until all the symptoms are gone.

After the bath, clean your nails. Then look for sores. Remove unhealthy scabs; they're a hiding place for staphylococcus bacteria. Gently clean out all pus from the sores, using a gauze pad. Then wash all pans and the tub with bleach or Lysol® or a good disinfectant, and wash your hands thoroughly with soap. Put on fresh clothes once a day. Then apply one of the following.

Comfrey. This is good for staph because it draws out the infection. Any of the methods described under Cuts, Wounds, and Sores (see Index) can be used. This is the most popular remedy for staph.

Burdock. Use the leaves and apply as with comfrey. Burdock is also drawing and is excellent for the skin. It can also be combined with comfrey leaf, using equal proportions of each.

Bacitracin or Neosporin. Some cases of staph are too advanced to respond well to herbal treatments. Don't torture yourself; a prolonged battle with an infectious disease will wear down your body's resistance far more rapidly than the use of an antibiotic ointment. These are both cheap, topical ointments that are available in most drugstores without a prescription. Apply to the sores 1 to 3 times a day after soaking. Continue to use the other remedies as well.

Internal Treatments

Vitamin C. Take 250 to 1000 mg. of vitamin C, 3 times a day, to detoxify the body. Drink juices and teas freely. In addition, use one or both of the following remedies.

Oil Of Bitter Orange. This remedy is used by naturopaths for staph, and I've seen it clear up boils that would not respond even to antibiotics. Bitter oranges grow in Africa, and they are too strong to eat. The oil is very powerful. Take 4 drops in about 1/2 cup of orange juice 3 times a day (3 drops for children). Use until all symptoms are gone, and then for another 2 to 3 days. Most cases clear up with one 1/4-ounce bottle in 3 to 7 days, but if it's a long-standing case, you may need up to 3 bottles. This remedy is available in some herb and health food stores, or you can order it from Nature's Herbs (see Resources).

Echinacea and Burdock Tea. Burdock has a bitter flavor. Drink 1 cup, 3 times a day until symptoms are gone, and then 1 cup per day for another 3 days.

Recipe: Echinacea and Burdock Tea. Bring 4 cups of water to a boil and add 2 teaspoons echinacea root and 2 teaspoons burdock root. Cover and simmer for 20 minutes.

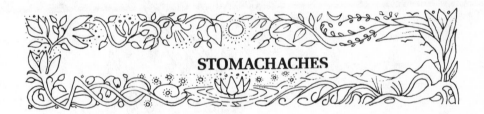

STOMACHACHES

The stomach is often confused with the intestines. The stomach is located at the center and left side of the body, above the navel and below the diaphragm. The small intestines, located just below the navel, is where most digestion takes place. This is where most people indicate when they say their stomach hurts.

The most commonly mentioned causes of stomachaches are overeating; eating too fast; eating when upset, nervous, tense, or anxious; and eating bad food combinations, especially combining fruits and vegetables.

Mint and chamomile teas are both helpful, whether the pain comes from the stomach or the small intestines. These teas can be taken separately or combined. They work for stomachaches, stomach cramps, upset stomach after meals, and overeating.

Mint Tea. Peppermint, spearmint, alfalfa/mint, and catnip are all effective.

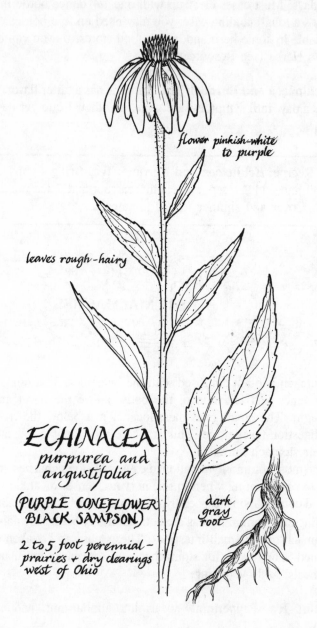

flower pinkish-white
to purple

leaves rough-hairy

ECHINACEA
purpurea and
angustifolia

(PURPLE CONEFLOWER
BLACK SAMPSON)

2 to 5 foot perennial –
prairies + dry clearings
west of Ohio

dark
gray
root

> **Recipe: Mint or Chamomile Tea.** Make a strong brew using 2
> teaspoons of either herb per cup of boiling water. Steep for 5 minutes.
> Use the fresh herb if you have it (4 teaspoons per cup). Drink 1 cup
> of tea and wait 15 minutes to 1 hour. If you are not all better, have
> another cup. Repeat as needed.

When to See a Medical Worker

Consult a medical worker any time the pain is severe, persistent, or increasing over several hours. The cause of abdominal pain is often difficult to diagnose and can be quite serious.

Be sure to consult a health care provider if the pain localizes in one particular area, if there is bleeding from the bowel, other than slight streaks on the toilet paper, if there has been a recent injury to the abdomen, or if the feces are black. If the pain is worse after a meal, it could be a duodenal ulcer. If there is any possibility of an ectopic pregnancy (implantation in the fallopian tube rather than the uterus), there would be severe pain on one side of the abdomen and vaginal bleeding. If the pain begins around the navel or just below the breast bone and then later settles in the lower right area of the pelvis, suspect appendicitis. If home-canned foods or meats that have been improperly refrigerated have been consumed within the last 36 hours, suspect botulism.

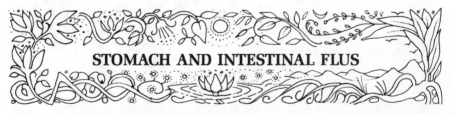

STOMACH AND INTESTINAL FLUS

When there's a virus in the digestive system, there may be nausea, vomiting, diarrhea, cramps, and loss of interest in food. There may also be headaches and fever. The flu usually goes away by itself within 24 to 48 hours, but a dose of slippery elm, cinnamon, golden seal, and cayenne almost always works within 10 minutes. This is the remedy that makes the most skeptical people say, "You converted me!"

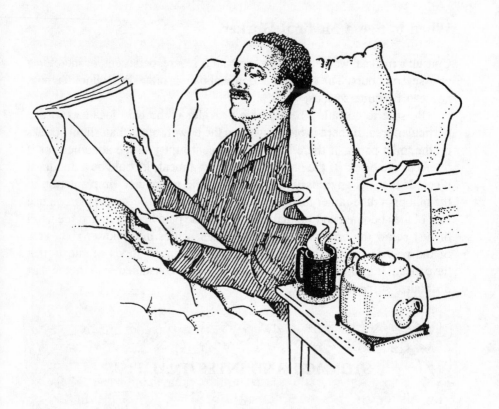

When your stomach hurts so badly that you just want to curl up in a ball, take 1 or 2 of these caps. They're just the thing for when your kid wakes up in the morning and says, "My tummy hurts. I don't want to go to school." Just give them 1 or 2 caps and then wait 10 minutes. When they're feeling better, put a couple more in their pocket and send them off to school.

It's a good idea to have some of these stomach capsules already prepared, because when you are feeling sick and nauseated, you may not have the patience to prepare them.

Golden seal—like garlic—is reputed to have antibiotic properties and may destroy beneficial intestinal bacteria. For this reason, I suggest taking 100 mg. vitamin C for detoxification and 2 to 3 tablespoons of plain yogurt 1 or 2 hours after taking golden seal. Continue to take the yogurt 3 times a day for 3 days after finishing treatment with golden seal. This helps to restore the beneficial intestinal bacteria. (See also Index: Nausea; Vomiting.)

Recipe: Slippery Elm, Cinnamon, Golden Seal, and Cayenne Capsules. Combine 1 teaspoon slippery elm powder, 1 teaspoon cinnamon powder, 1 teaspoon golden seal powder, and 1 teaspoon cayenne powder. Mix thoroughly. Fill empty 00 gelatin capsules (available in most drugstores), which hold 1/4 teaspoon each. Take 1 to 2 caps and follow with 1/2 cup warm water.

Or put 1/4 teaspoon of the mixture on a butter knife and drop it on the back of your tongue and swallow quickly with warm water (it's hot and bitter, but there aren't many taste buds on the back of your tongue).

Take 1 or 2 capsules (or butter knife doses) before each meal, or less, as needed. One or 2 doses are usually enough, but it can be continued for days if necessary. If there is vomiting, just use the slippery elm and cinnamon, because the taste of golden seal and cayenne can be very unpleasant when it comes back on you. Some people (including many children) are sensitive to cayenne, so if there's a burning in the stomach, give milk as an antidote and then omit cayenne from future doses.

When to Call a Medical Worker

If the symptoms are severe, consider the possibility of dysentery or food poisoning, and contact a medical worker.

Suspect botulism if home-canned foods or meats that have been inadequately refrigerated have been consumed within the last 36 hours.

With vomiting and diarrhea, there is danger of dehydration. When the body loses a lot of fluid, the cells begin to take back the fluid from the blood. This can eventually cause the blood vessels to collapse in vascular shock, which is fatal.

Touch the tongue and membranes of the mouth every hour or so before giving fluids. If there is dry, sticky saliva (i.e., if this doesn't leave a wet spot on your finger), call a doctor.

If you see dark, concentrated urine, consult a doctor. In a baby, this means a diaper that's less wet than usual. If you suspect dehydration, write down how many times urinations occur in each 8-hour period. If the number of urinations get smaller, this is cause for concern.

If the temperature is 103° or higher or the pulse is higher than normal, consult a doctor. Take the pulse by holding the second or third finger of one hand to the blood vessel on the inside wrist of the other hand. Use a watch that indicates seconds, and time how many pulsations occur in a 30-second period. Multiply this by 2, and you'll have the pulse rate. Take the pulse 2 or 3 times a day, and note if it becomes faster than normal (see Index: Pulse rates).

Consult a doctor if vomiting and diarrhea continue and fluid can't be held down for 10 to 12 hours in an adult or child over 10 years; for 10 hours in a child 6 to 10 years old; for 8 hours in a child 2 to 6 years old; or for 6 hours in a child under 2 years old.

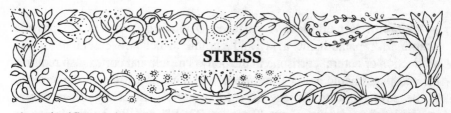

STRESS

Any significant change will produce the physiological symptoms of stress. Whether it's the severe stress caused by the death of a close family member, or the relatively mild stress of a Christmas holiday, whenever we have to change our daily routine it causes the same reaction: the hypothalamus at the base of the brain produces a substance that stimulates the pituitary gland. The pituitary secretes ACTH which travels through the blood to the two adrenal glands (which sit on top of the kidneys). They secrete corticoids which prepare the body for "fight or flight."

We can meet stress with either adaptation or resistance. Children are highly adaptable and emotionally expressive, so they get over stress quickly. The older we get, the more rigid we tend to become. When we lose our powers of adaptation, we experience exhaustion.

I have found that the best way to adapt to stress is through emotional release. Whenever we're under unusual stress, if we can find a way to express our feelings, this helps to alleviate the pressure. Stress is normal, but when it builds up, it becomes distress.

Stress and illness are characterized by the following syndrome:

1. Proteins are drawn from the thymus and lymph glands and broken down to form blood sugar for energy. If the stress continues for a long time, these glands shrink, less white blood cells are produced, and the body's self-defense system is weakened.

2. Blood pressure increases.

3. Minerals are drawn from the bones. This explains why you get an aching feeling in your bones when you are sick.

4. Fat is mobilized from fatty tissues, which is why continued stress can cause peptic ulcers.

5. Salt is retained. People under continuous stress tend to look "puffy," especially in the face. There is often edema and weight gain.

If your diet is good, you can experience periods of stress without harm. But during periods of extreme stress, supplement your diet in order to avoid nervousness and illness. Whenever you are under stress, take supplements of vitamins B and C. If the stress increases, also take vitamins A and E.

Vitamin B Complex. A balanced B vitamin complex will provide vitamin B2, pantothenic acid, and choline which are essential for the production of natural cortisone in the body. The adrenal cortex also requires B2 and pantothenic acid. The dosage will vary according to the severity of the stress, but an average dose for a person under significant stress is a tablet that contains about 10 mg. of B2, B3, and B6 3 times a day or a tablet that contains 25 to 50 mg. once a day.

Vitamin C. This vitamin is essential to the functioning of the adrenal cortex. During times of severe stress, be sure to take at least 250 mg. 3 times a day. Ascorbic acid is less expensive than the natural forms of vitamin C and is adequate for treating stress.

Vitamin E. This vitamin is more concentrated in the pituitary gland than in any other part of the body. It prevents the pituitary and adrenal hormones from being destroyed by oxygen. An average dose for times of stress is 400 I.U. once a day. (See precautions concerning taking vitamin E in chapter 5.)

Vitamin A. This vitamin is important for the optimum functioning of the adrenal cortex. A healthy dose is 10,000 I.U. a day.

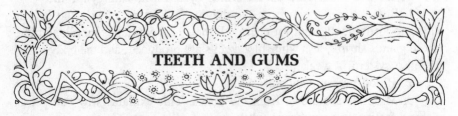

TEETH AND GUMS

Cavities are caused by plaque, which is a yellowish-white film made up of food debris and bacteria. It converts sugar into acid, and the acid dissolves away the enamel of the tooth. Then it penetrates to the softer second layer—the dentine—where it spreads more easily. If untreated, it will spread to the pulp area where the nerves and blood vessels are. The bone may become infected, and an abscess may form. Then a root canal becomes necessary.

If this plaque is removed once every 24 to 36 hours, then decay cannot set in. But if it is not removed, it can harden into calculus, which can only be removed by a special cleaning.

When gums are healthy, they don't bleed when brushed. At the point of contact between the gums and the visible part of the teeth, there are pockets where the brush can penetrate, called the sulcus. A healthy sulcus is 1 to 3 mm. deep.

Gum disease is caused when plaque accumulates in the pockets. Then the gums become swollen and will bleed when brushed and flossed. The gums will spread away from the teeth and the pockets will become deeper. The plaque will harden into calculus (it only takes about a week), which further irritates the gums. The pockets continue to deepen until the plaque reaches the bones which support the teeth. Then the teeth become loose. The bone recedes, and this damage is irreversible. The only recourse then is to remove the tooth.

But all this can be prevented by proper care of the teeth and gums on a daily basis. If you've been neglecting your mouth, don't be surprised if flossing and brushing cause your gums to bleed. This is a sign that you need to do this, and the more regularly you floss, the healthier your gums and teeth will become, and then the bleeding will stop.

The best method of brushing is to use a soft brush and hold it at an angle, so that the bristles splay out and reach into the pockets between the gums and the teeth. Position the brush and then gently vibrate it in place. Then move the brush to the next position and vibrate it again. This method cleans the teeth, the pockets, and also stimulates the gums.

Most decay and gum disease occurs mainly between the teeth, where the brush cannot reach. Flossing is the most effective way of cleaning these areas. See your dentist for a demonstration of how to floss. Remember to floss at least once a day.

Toothaches

If you have a toothache, see a dentist as soon as possible. Meanwhile, here are some good relief measures.

Niacin. Take 50 to 100 mg. of niacin. Some people get a niacin rush: a flushing of the face and a prickly sensation at the extremities or all over the body. Don't panic; it will pass shortly. The niacin usually relieves the pain entirely. Niacin can also be taken as niacinamide with the rest of the B complex and will cause no reaction.

Garlic. Place a piece of garlic in your mouth behind the painful tooth, for about an hour.

Oil of Cloves. This is a well-known anesthetic. Soak a plug of cotton in the oil and then insert the cotton directly into the cavity.

Gingivitis, Periodontitus, and Trench Mouth

If you have gum problems, here are some home remedies to try.

Hydrogen Peroxide Rinse. This is excellent for bleeding gums, sores in the mouth, and trench mouth. Combine 1/4 cup hydrogen peroxide and 1/4 cup water. Rinse the mouth and swish through the teeth 3 times, 3 times a day, for 5 days.

Golden Seal and Myrrh. This tastes bitter, but it will do wonders to strengthen the gums. Combine equal parts of golden seal powder and myrrh powder and use to brush the teeth and gums, 3 or 4 times a day.

Preparation for Dental Work

When you see a dentist to have several fillings done, or to have a tooth pulled, or to have a root canal, you put your body through a lot of stress. If you prepare yourself for the experience by taking the vitamins described under Stress and the Rescue Remedy (see Index), you will reduce the pain and tension considerably, and this will speed up the healing process.

Preparation for Root Canal

When there is an infection at the root of a tooth, it is usually treated by a root canal. First the infection has to be treated, and this is generally done with antibiotics. There is an alternative. Sometimes the root canal tooth pack provides total relief, and sometimes it just provides temporary relief until you can get to the dentist.

> **Recipe: Root Canal Tooth Pack.** Combine 1 part golden seal, 3 parts comfrey root, 3 parts bayberry bark, and 3 parts white oak bark. If you cannot obtain one or two of these herbs, just use the ones you can get. Add enough water to make it into a thick paste and pack on the cheek side of the tooth, near the root. For best results, wrap the herbs in cheesecloth and use a few stitches to hold it together. Moisten with a few drops of hot water. Apply just before going to bed. Repeat for 6 nights, then rest the seventh. Repeat as long as necessary. (This recipe comes from Dr. John R. Christopher.)

After a Root Canal

To minimize the trauma of a root canal, take 3 garlic cloves a day and 1000 mg. vitamin C 3 times a day to prevent infection. Take 4 tablets of 6X potency homeopathic arnica for pain (see Index). Apply the root canal tooth pack (as described above) to take down the swelling. This routine is very effective and should restore you to normal within a day or two.

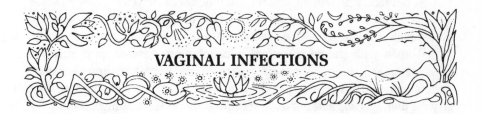

VAGINAL INFECTIONS

Vaginal infections are experienced by almost every woman at some time, and by a surprising number of women almost all the time. The vagina normally secretes a small amount of clear or milky discharge, which becomes heavier during ovulation. A vaginal infection is characterized by an offensive odor, itchiness, and excessive discharge. Sometimes there is discomfort or itchiness during or just after intercourse.

Many women believe that recurrent outbreaks of vaginal infections relate to how they feel about their bodies, or about birth control, or about their sexual partners. Guilt about sex, confusion about the role a woman should take in bed, or lack of enthusiasm for one's lover (which may involve inter-course without proper lubrication, which is irritating) are factors that seem to contribute to recurrent outbreaks of vaginal infections. When these issues are dealt with—sometimes with the help of a therapist, doctor, or friend—the infections often go away.

Normally, glucose (blood sugar) is exuded from the blood serum into the vagina to keep it moist. The friendly organisms that grow in the vagina metabolize the glucose and the by-product is lactic acid. This creates an acidic environment in the vagina that prevents infections. This environment can be disturbed by the hormonal changes that occur during pregnancy, by stress, and by taking antibiotics, among other things. Observing a few general precautions may prevent a vaginal infection from starting.

Wear cotton underpants, or none at all. Try to avoid leotards and tights made of synthetics, which provide the perfect warm, moist environment for the growth of yeast.

Wipe from front to back after a bowel movement. Don't share wash-cloths or towels. Avoid soap, because it's alkaline. Avoid commercial douches or frequent douches of any kind which wash away the beneficial natural secretions. Avoid feminine hygiene deodorants. A good substitute is a tablet of acidophilus or yogurt inserted into the vagina before going to bed at night. These are available in most drugstores and health food stores.

Minimize sugar, sweets, and refined foods because yeast grows on sugar. Get enough rest so you don't feel tired in the morning. Make sure your diet is adequate in vitamins A, B, and C. Minimize stress.

Women with stubborn vaginal infections may have an overgrowth of *candida* (yeast) throughout their system. A naturopath or knowledgeable doctor can determine if you have *candida* and can explain how to treat it with diet, garlic, acidophilus, and possibly antifungal medication. For more information, read *Back to Health* by Dennis Remington, M.D.

If you don't know what kind of infection you have, try the garlic sup-pository or acidolphilus tablets as described below.

Preventive Cleanliness

Washing the vagina with clear running water can be an effective way to prevent vaginitis. The natural acid secretions provide the perfect chemistry for cleansing and purifying the vagina. Anything that changes this acidic climate makes a woman more vulnerable to infection. This explains why acid substances, like vinegar, are used in the treatment of vaginitis. The opposite of acid is alkaline, so anything that is alkaline is potentially disruptive inside the vagina. This includes semen, menstrual fluid, lochia (the blood flow after childbirth), and soap. Soap should never be used in the vagina. There are some expensive acid soaps, but why pay for what you already have? The natural acidic discharge from the vagina is self-cleansing. A healthy woman only needs to wash with plain water regularly and after each time she has intercourse (it doesn't have to be immediately after). If there is an infection or irritation, a daily wash with a vinegar rinse is advisable.

Vinegar Rinse. Add 2 teaspoons white vinegar (don't use apple cider vinegar because it may ferment) to 1 cup water. Squat in the bathtub or over a large bowl. It is not necessary to remove clothes that can be kept above the waist. You may want to close the drain on the tub and run a little warm water so it won't be cold to your feet. Dip your finger into the vinegar solution and then insert it into your vagina and move it around inside. Remove your finger and you may see a white discharge. Then rinse your finger under the tap or in another bowl of fresh water. Repeat this several times, or until the discharge is gone. The whole process only takes a few minutes.

Encourage your partner to wash after intercourse. Uncircumcised men are more likely to be carriers of vaginal infections. This could be indicated by little red spots on the foreskin. Men can also wash with a solution of 2 teaspoons of white vinegar in 1 cup of water.

When treating vaginal infections, try to avoid intercourse, which irritates the fragile vaginal tissues and introduces alkaline semen to the area. If you do have intercourse, ask your partner to use a condom and always make sure there is plenty of lubrication. Cocoa oil or vegetable oil make a good lubricant, as does a strong tea made of slippery elm. Add 2 tablespoons of slippery elm powder to 1 cup of boiling water. Simmer for 10 minutes.

Garlic Suppositories. If you start to get the symptoms of vaginitis (offensive odor, itch, excessive discharge), and you are sure you don't have a venereal disease (gonorrhea, syphilis), you can usually get rid of the infection by immediately treating with garlic. You don't even have to know what kind of infection you are harboring because garlic is effective for all kinds, particularly if it is used in the early stages.

Prepare a garlic suppository by carefully peeling one small or medium-size clove of garlic. Dip it in vegetable oil (to prevent burning) and insert it into the vagina like a tampon. It can be easily removed, like a diaphragm, by inserting your finger behind it and popping it out.

Remove the garlic every 12 hours and insert a fresh clove. Do this for 3 to 5 days. Don't be surprised if your discharge increases at first; this is the body's way of cleansing itself before the healing begins. However, if you experience a significant amount of burning or irritation, remove the garlic.

Yeast Infections

Yeast, also known as monilia, moniliasis, and *candida albicans,* is a fungus that normally grows in the vagina, rectum, and intestines. It may also grow on the skin, nails, mouth, lungs, and feet (where it is called athlete's foot). Overgrowth of yeast in the vagina is characterized by itching, unpleasant odor, irritation, and a whitish discharge that resembles cottage cheese.

Chronic yeast infections have been associated with the use of birth control pills. Yeast grows on sugar, so diabetic women and women who eat lots of sugar should have their urine tested for sugar. Pregnant women and women with high estrogen levels may also have trouble with yeast, because estrogen (which rises during pregnancy) cause the cells that line the uterus to produce more glycogen (sugar).

Garlic. Use as directed above.

Acidophilus. Lactobacillus acidophilus is a bacteria that grows naturally in the vagina, but can be wiped out by the use of broad-spectrum antibiotics, such as tetracycline and ampicillin. It ferments the vaginal secretions to make them acidic. Yeast also grows normally in the vagina, but when there is an overgrowth of yeast, a yeast infection occurs. Lactobacillus bulgaricus, or yogurt, is another form of the same bacteria.

Acidophilus comes in liquid and tablet form. The easiest method is to use acidophilus tablets. Insert 1 or 2 tablets in your vagina each night before going to bed. Alternatively, a rinse can be made with the liquid, using 2 teaspoons in 1 cup of water and applying it as with the vinegar rinse described above. The infection should clear up within 7 to 10 days. Both the liquid and the tablets can be obtained from drugstores and health food stores.

If the reason for the infection is the use of antibiotics, wait until you finish the antibiotics, then take 2 acidophilus tablets or 1 to 2 teaspoons liquid acidophilus by mouth about 1/2 hour before each meal for 1 week.

Yogurt. Lactobacillus bulgaricus ferments milk to make yogurt, just as the beneficial bacteria in the vagina ferment vaginal secretions to make them acidic. The easiest method is to insert 1 or 2 yogurt tablets into your vagina each night before going to bed. Alternatively, insert 1 to 2 tablespoons of plain, unsweetened yogurt with a vaginal applicator. Or dissolve 2 tablespoons of yogurt in 1 cup of warm water and use this as a rinse, applying it as with the vinegar rinse described earlier in this section. Whatever method is used, it should be repeated once a day for a week or twice a week until the infection is gone.

If the reason for the infection is the use of antibiotics, wait until you finish the antibiotics, then take 2 tablespoons of yogurt by mouth about 1/2 hour before each meal for about 1 week.

Vinegar Rinse. This remedy, as described earlier in this section, works best when used at the first sign of an infection. Some women like to rinse with vinegar each day and then insert an acidophilus pill each night for 1 week.

Golden Seal and Myrrh. A douche made of these two herbs is the remedy I usually recommend to women with chronic yeast infections who have tried the above remedies without success.

Cover 1 teaspoon of golden seal powder and 1 teaspoon of myrrh powder (or 2 teaspoons golden seal powder) with 1 quart boiling water and steep until comfortably cool. Douche with the liquid once a day for 3 days. If the infection is itchy, douche with the cool tea. Otherwise it can be warmed.

It is a good idea to also take golden seal internally. Fill size 00 gelatin capsules with golden seal and take 1 per day. Also take 2 tablespoons yogurt and 100 mg. of vitamin C to counteract any possible toxicity from the golden seal.

Vitamins. Several women with stubborn yeast infections have reported remarkable results from taking 100 mg. of B1, B2, B6, and 200 mg. of B3, as well as pantothenic acid and the rest of the complex, supplemented by foods rich in vitamin B. This high dosage of B vitamins should be taken for 2 months and then gradually discontinued. Pantothenic acid and B6 stimulate the production of antibodies and white blood cells.

Also take at least 1000 mg. of vitamin C a day to stop infections and render bacteria harmless, as well as inhibit the further growth of harmful bacteria. Take supplements of vitamins A and E for 3 days with meals. Vitamin A is vital to the health of mucous membranes, and vitamin E protects vitamin A.

Diet. Some women have observed that eating a lot of meat, dairy products, grains, or sugars (including honey) made their yeast infections worse. A diet of mostly fruits and vegetables for 2 to 3 weeks may rid you of a chronic yeast infection.

Treatment for Men. A woman with a recurring vaginal yeast infection needs the active participation of her partner to get rid of it. First the male partner must determine if he is a passive carrier or an active carrier of the yeast. A passive carrier has yeast on the skin and possibly on the pubic hairs or in the anus (a small amount of yeast grows naturally in the intestines and anus; a yeast infection occurs when there is an overgrowth of yeast). An active carrier has yeast in the urethra and re-infects his partner during intercourse. A medical worker uses a cotton swab to scrape the suspected area and examines it under a microscope.

If the yeast is on the surface only, and not in the urethra, both partners can wash thoroughly after (and preferably before) intercourse with 1 tablespoon white vinegar in 2 cups warm water. If the yeast is internal, the man should drink 3/4 cup of cranberry juice 3 times a day, or take 1 tablespoon of apple cider vinegar and 1 tablespoon honey in 1/2 to 1 cup of hot water 2 times a day, or take 3000 mg. of vitamin C per day to acidify his urine, which should clear out the yeast.

It is also important, while the infection is active, to use a condom or to avoid genital intercourse altogether. This will help prevent re-infections.

Trichomoniasis (Trichomonas)

This infection is caused by a microscopic protozoa with a tail (*Trichomonas vaginalis*). Women who have trichomonas experience a yellow to yellowish-green discharge, itching, burning, and a fishy odor. Symptoms may be worse before and after menstrual periods. Men are usually asymptomatic, though men are carriers, and it can be passed during sexual contact. An uncircumcised man may have little red spots on his foreskin.

The standard treatment is Flagyl, but Flagyl has caused gene mutations and birth defects and cancer in animals.

Unfortunately, herbal alternatives for trichomonas are among the least impressive home remedies. None of them are more than 50 percent effective. This is not surprising since only extremely potent medications are effective in killing off this stubborn bug. Nevertheless, since Flagyl is so harmful, it is certainly worth trying a home remedy first.

It has been found that spermicidal jellies (the kind used with diaphragms) inhibit the growth of trichomoniasis and possibly yeast. Some women who are very susceptible to trichomonas infections (for example, women who use birth control pills) have found that using spermicidal jelly once every 2 weeks can prevent trich. Jelly can be inserted into the vagina with a foam applicator, available in drugstores.

A trichomonas infection can cause a bladder infection. During intercourse, the protozoa can move out of the vaginal opening and into the urethral opening.

Trichomonas is a protozoa that spreads easily, so hygiene is an essential part of the treatment. All bedding and clothing should be laundered, hands should be washed after any contact with the genitals, and the toilet seat should be cleaned with a bleach solution after each use, until the infection has cleared up.

Garlic Suppository. Use as directed earlier in this section. A variation (which may be slightly more successful) is to douche with 1 tablespoon white vinegar in 1 quart of warm water every 24 hours, when you remove the garlic clove. Douche every second day for 1 week with a combination of 1 tablespoon golden seal root (powder is okay), 1 teaspoon witch hazel leaves, and 1 teaspoon comfrey root. Add the herbs to 4 cups of water and simmer for 20 minutes. Let cool, then use as the douche.

Aloe Vera Suppository. Cut a section from the leaf of an aloe plant that is 2 inches long and 1/2 inch wide. Remove the outer skin and you will have a piece of aloe that works well as a suppository. Insert it directly into your vagina. This will help relieve the itchy, burning feeling. It will dissolve or come out by itself. If you don't have an aloe plant, you can use aloe vera gel by inserting 1 to 2 tablespoons with a foam applicator. Use every other day for the first week, then twice a week for the second week.

Chaparrel and Chamomile. Make a douche by covering one handful of chaparrel (*Larrea tridentata*) and 1 handful of chamomile with 1 quart of boiling water. Let steep for 10 minutes, then cool. Douche 2 to 3 times a week for 2 weeks.

Treatments for Men. This organism is usually killed off in the man by avoiding ejaculation for 10 days. Apparently the protozoa are nourished by semen. But there are stubborn cases where the trichomonads survive in the prostate and seminal vesicles, so be sure to get checked by a medical worker after 10 days to be certain you've gotten rid of the organism. It is also advisable to get plenty of rest, a good diet, and to eat 1 clove of raw garlic a day.

Hemophilus

The symptoms of *Hemophilus vaginalis* are similar to those of trichomonas, although the discharge may be creamy white or grayish and particularly foul-smelling after intercourse. It is transmitted primarily through sexual intercourse, so your partner must be treated also. The treatment for men is the same as for trichomonas, as described above.

Garlic and Vinegar. Alternate the garlic suppository (described earlier in this section) with the vinegar rinse (described earlier in this section) from night to night for 1 to 2 weeks, until the symptoms disappear. Some individuals have had good results with garlic suppositories alone for 5 days.

Nonspecific Vaginitis

This is a term used for vaginal infections other than yeast, trichomonas, and *Hemophilus*. About 90 percent of what used to be called nonspecific is now recognized as hemophilus.

Nonspecific vaginitis may be characterized by a white or yellow or possibly bloody discharge. There may be lower back pain, cramps, and swollen glands in the abdomen and inner thighs. The treatment is to use garlic suppositories and a douche of chamomile and chaparrel as described earlier in this section.

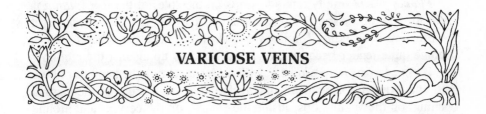

VARICOSE VEINS

Walking and exercising provides the best prevention for varicose veins. The veins flow through muscles and during exercise the muscles contract, which assists blood return. Elevation of the legs is beneficial in collapsing the veins, giving them a rest. Likewise, placing the chest lower than the hips by getting down on your elbows and knees allows better drainage for the veins of the legs. A daily dose of at least 100 mg. of vitamin C will help to keep your veins healthy and elastic.

The underlying cause of varicose veins tends to be a secret desire to kick somebody. Vigorously kicking a pillow relieves tension and gives the leg exercise at the same time. This can be quite effective. Try using a big pillow, and put it up against the wall in a corner of the room. If you can give yourself permission to release your emotions in the privacy of your own room, you won't harm anyone else, and you'll probably feel a lot better.

Vitamin E. This vitamin helps eliminate varicose veins. Take 400 to 800 I.U. per day. (See chapter 5 for precautions concerning taking vitamin E.)

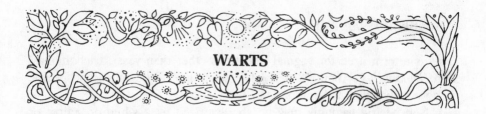

WARTS

Warts are small, hard, abnormal growths on the skin or adjoining mucous membrane, caused by a virus. Half of these warts will go away by themselves, without treatment. Warts are more common among young people. Most warts are less than 1/4 inch in diameter; they may be flat, raised, dry, or moist. They are usually flesh colored, or darker than the skin.

Plantar warts simply refers to warts on the soles of the feet (*planta* is Latin for sole of the foot). These warts become very sensitive because of the pressure of walking. Similarly, warts on the knees or elbows tend to become quite tender because they frequently rub up against the clothing.

Venereal warts (*condyloma acuminatum*) appear on the genitals of both men and women. On women, they're found at the bottom of the vaginal opening, on the vaginal lips, inside the vagina, on the cervix, and around the anus. On a man, they occur toward the tip of the penis, sometimes under the foreskin, on the shaft of the penis, or on the scrotum. When small, they look like hard raised skin, but when large they take on a cauliflower appearance. Warmth and moisture encourage their growth. They are caused by a virus, and they're contagious, so sexual contact does spread them, though they can occur without contact. They will appear 1 to 3 months after contact, and they don't hurt. If you are treating yourself for venereal warts, make sure that your partner gets treated at the same time. If the warts are only on the penis or inside the vagina, then using a condom can help prevent their spreading. Vitamin E has been effective for venereal warts, and vitamin A has been used in the same way. Of course, don't use a band-aid for venereal warts; just apply the oil directly to the warts.

Vitamin E. Open a capsule of vitamin E oil and squeeze the oil onto a band-aid, then apply the band-aid to the warts and leave it on for 24 hours, then replace it with a new band-aid, also with vitamin E oil. The warts should diminish and then disappear within 2 to 6 weeks. Note: The capsule may be any size or strength, from 100 I.U. to 800 I.U.

Castor Oil. Castor oil is available in drugstores. Dab a little oil on the warts at least 2 to 3 times a day and just before going to bed at night. You can use a band-aid as as described above. The warts should begin to decrease in size within a week, and they're usually gone within 2 to 3 months.

Milkweed. Cover the warts with the milky sap of this plant several times a day. The warts should be gone within 2 to 6 weeks.

Asparagus. This remedy has worked in some case where none of the above were effective. For best results, combine it with one of the above remedies. Get a can of asparagus (or fresh or frozen) and put the juice and the asparagus in a blender, or just mash it up with a potato masher or fork. Take 4 tablespoons of the puree morning and evening. The warts should dry up and peel off within 1 to 2 months. This has been especially effective in cases where there were many warts in one area of the body.

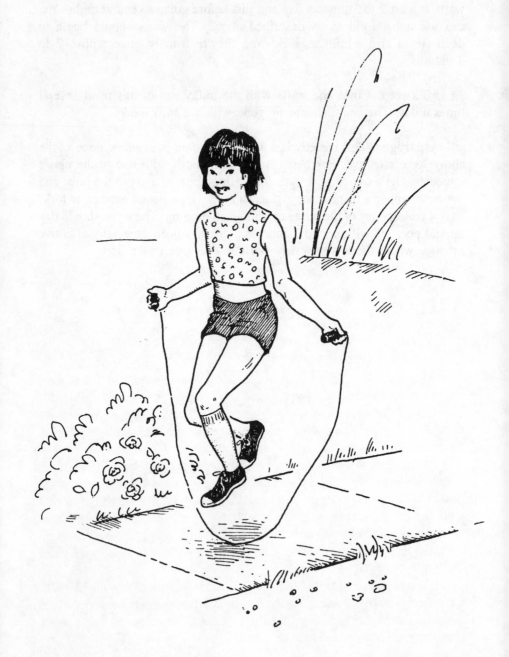

Chapter 3

Remedies for Infants and Children

In this chapter are remedies and advice that deals with some of the special health care needs of infants and children. For such common complaints as colds, insect bites, burns, cuts, and other problems that affect adults as well, see chapter 2. Some of these problems, such as hiccups and nosebleeds, are also experienced by adults, and the same remedies can be used.

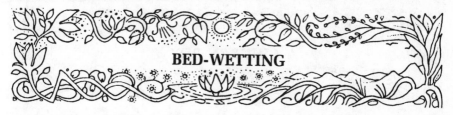

BED-WETTING

It is normal for kids to wet their beds, but by the time they are 3 to 6 years old, most of them have stopped. Yet a surprising number of children—especially boys—continue to have "accidents" or simply have no control at night for many years. This causes a great deal of embarrassment, particularly if they want to spend the night at a friend's house.

Bed-wetting is a great inconvenience to the parent who must wash the bedclothes every day. One cause of bed-wetting is suppressed anger toward one or both parents—a way of saying, "Piss on you!" It may help to find a counselor or therapist who can help the child to express his or her anger or resentment. On the other hand, some children simply have weak bladders and they sleep very soundly. In any case, try not to make your child feel guilty.

It is reasonable to expect that a child who is 8 years old or older should take responsibility for removing the wet bedclothes and putting on dry ones.

These remedies have been helpful to many children, particularly when they themselves have a desire to stop.

Strengthening the Sphincter Muscles. When the child urinates, have the child stop midstream once or twice. This teaches control of the muscle and strengthens it, making it easier for a child to "hold it in" at night.

A problem that is common among children who wet their beds is that they dream of going to the bathroom. Sphincter control can be helpful here, too, because children can be taught to always urinate just a tiny bit before they let out the full stream. If they continue this habit even in their sleep, then the experience of getting a little wet may be enough to convince them that they are, in fact, dreaming, and should get up to go to the bathroom.

Acupressure. Apply firm but gentle pressure with the fingernail to the lines at the inside of the two joints of both of the child's little fingers. Do this for 15 to 30 seconds at each joint before bedtime. Children can learn to do this for themselves.

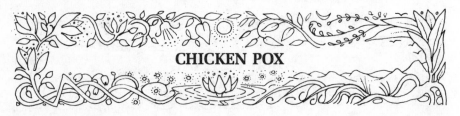

CHICKEN POX

This is a common childhood disease that is rarely serious and does not occur more than once. Children are very contagious from 2 days before the rash appears until all the sores dry up (1 to 2 weeks later). The incubation period is 2 to 3 weeks (a child may get the disease and not show any symptoms for 2 to 3 weeks).

The earliest symptoms of chicken pox are a slight headache, fever, backache, and loss of appetite. After a day or two, small, flat red spots appear, usually on the chest and back. Within a few hours, these become raised, and they resemble pimples or blisters. After another day or two, the blisters break and the sores form a crust or scab, which peels off in 5 to 20 days. The scab causes severe itching. There may be only a few sores, or there may be hundreds. The eruptions of new sores may last from 2 to 6 days. The fever usually goes away by the time all the sores have formed crusts. With some children, the symptoms are so mild that the disease goes unnoticed. *Note:* Adults do not get chicken pox, but the same virus that causes chicken pox also causes herpes zoster (shingles).

Chicken pox are usually treated at home, but if the sores become infected or do not heal properly, see a medical worker. Call ahead, in order not to infect other children in the doctor's office. Make every effort to isolate your child until all the sores form scabs. However, exposure to siblings is hard to avoid, and over 90 percent of brothers and sisters do catch it. It is spread by droplets from the mouth or throat, or by direct contact with the blisters, or by contaminated clothing.

To reduce the fever that comes with chicken pox, see the discussion on Fevers in chapter 2 (see Index). If the fever goes above 103°, consult a medical worker. Encephalitis, which is characterized by a high fever, is a dangerous complication of chicken pox.

The main problem with chicken pox is the itching and then the scratching, which irritates and spreads the sores and can cause scarring. Comfrey paste has been extremely effective in minimizing itching and keeping the outbreak mild.

Comfrey Paste. Make a paste by combining 1/4 cup honey and 1/4 cup wheat germ oil in a blender. While the machine is running, add fresh chopped comfrey leaves, fresh chopped comfrey root, and dried comfrey root powder until the mixture has the thickness of a paste. Apply freely to sores. (Don't use dried whole comfrey root in your blender; it could break the blades). Most health food stores carry some form of comfrey ointment, which is also effective.

Baking Soda Baths. This is a time-honored remedy for relieving the itch of chicken pox. Add 1/2 cup of baking soda to a warm bath by sprinkling it under the running water. Such baths can be taken frequently. They are helpful, but less impressive than comfrey paste.

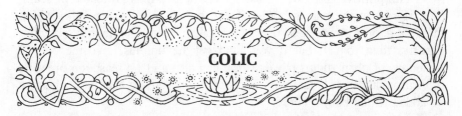

COLIC

Colic is a pain in the abdomen caused by spasms of the intestine, and it is most common in infants 3 months and younger. Colic is often caused by too much gas. If your baby is irritable every day, in a regular pattern, and if the infant's legs are drawn up, or the abdomen feels hard, or the feet or hands are tightly clenched, chances are the baby is suffering from colic. Colic should also be suspected if the baby cries loudly, turns red in the face, and expels gas from the anus or belches it from the stomach. Excess gas may be caused by the baby swallowing too much air, drinking too fast or too frequently, or from overexcitement.

It's helpful to provide a quiet, secure environment for both the mother and child, particularly before and at feeding time. A baby is sensitive to its parent's moods, so try to keep calm and don't worry too much when your baby has colic. A calming tea, such as catnip, is useful for the parents, as well as the child. (Recipe below.)

If the baby is nursing, it may be nursing too often, which doesn't give the milk enough time to digest. If you find yourself offering the breast every time your baby cries, consider other alternatives.

Babies who are given cow's milk sometimes get colic. Cow's milk is a very complex protein, difficult for the human body to break down. Cow's milk has only half as much lactose as human milk. Lactose encourages the growth of lactobacillus, a helpful flora that aids in digestion and assimilation. Without lactobacillus, there is likely to be more gas, so cow's milk makes a baby more vulnerable to colic.

Some infants are so sensitive to cow's milk that they develop colic if they are breast-feeding and their mothers drink it. If you are nursing and your baby has colic, try eliminating cow's milk from your diet. If the colic disappears within 1 or 2 days, and then comes back within a day of reintroducing cow's milk, you will know this is the cause of the colic. *Goat's milk* is more easily digested than cow's milk. Add acidophilus as explained below.

Acidophilus. Add 1 or 2 teaspoons of acidophilus (available in health food stores) to the baby's bottle (it can be added to goat's milk, which makes a good formula, tea, or juice or taken plain). Acidophilus is more effective than yogurt, but if you can't get acidophilus, give the baby 2 teaspoons of plain yogurt per day. You can also add 1/4 teaspoon brewer's or torula yeast and 1/3 teaspoon molasses (this is also a laxative). This can be added to the baby's bottle.

Catnip Tea. This is a time-honored remedy for indigestion and gas, and it is soothing to the nerves. Give as needed.

> **Recipe: Catnip Tea.** Cover 1 teaspoon catnip with 1 cup boiling water and steep in a covered container for 5 minutes.

Slippery Elm Tea. This is my favorite remedy for colic and gas. It's also mildly laxative, so don't use it if the child has diarrhea. Bring 2 cups of water to a boil, sprinkle in 1 teaspoon of powdered or granulated slippery elm, simmer for 20 minutes, and strain. Begin with about 2 tablespoons (2 ounces) and refrigerate the rest. Wait 12 hours to see what effect it has on the colic and on the bowels. Increase the amount gradually, if necessary; it can be taken as much and as often as desired, provided it doesn't cause much diarrhea.

Peppermint Tea. Peppermint is not specific for colic, but if catnip and slippery elm are not available, peppermint is also good for the stomach, the nerves, for gas, and for spasms. Prepare as with catnip tea (above).

Burping. Remember that burping helps to relieve gas. The bounce-'n'-pat technique is usually the most reliable: Bounce your baby on your knees, put the baby back on your shoulder and pat on the back. Some babies like to be pounded rather vigorously—of course, don't do anything that hurts the baby or causes crying. Babies should be burped each time they finish nursing. If you do hold the baby on your shoulder, you may want to put a clean diaper on your shoulder first, because they usually spit up when they burp.

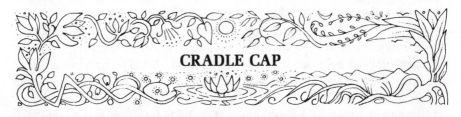

CRADLE CAP

This is an oily yellowish crust that sometimes occurs on the scalp of infants or small children. It is caused by the oversecretion of the sweat glands of the scalp.

Apply wheat germ oil, vitamin E oil, or cold-pressed vegetable oil and leave it on overnight. The next morning, gently scratch off the softened crust, or comb with a fine tooth comb. Then wash the baby's head with shampoo. Repeat in a few days if necessary.

If this method is not adequate, there may be a deficiency of vitamins A and B, which prevents the liver from metabolizing fats properly. Evaluate your own diet if you are nursing, or the baby's diet if you are not. Consider giving a vitamin supplement until the condition clears up.

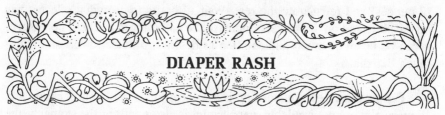

DIAPER RASH

A diaper rash can be an allergic reaction to a food that either the child eats or a nursing mother eats. If you are nursing and your baby has a persistent rash, try eliminating homogenized cow's milk from your diet for a week. If the rash goes away, try reintroducing cow's milk. It the rash returns within a day or two, then it is probably an allergy to cow's milk. You may want to try the same experiment with raw milk or goat's milk.

If the rash is not due to an allergy, the diaper may be causing the problem. If you are using paper diapers, try cloth diapers without rubber pants to let the air circulate. There are several brands of wool and cotton diaper covers, including BioBottoms and Nicki's. *Cornstarch* is an excellent powder to use to absorb moisture in the diaper. Dust it on the baby's bottom to soothe raw and tender skin.

If you are already using cloth diapers, try changing your detergent. Even Ivory is irritating to some babies. Basic H (available through Shaklee distributors) is a good soap for washing diapers. Avoid using ammonia and bleach, or if you do, rinse the diapers twice. Add 2 tablespoons of vinegar to the rinse water.

Sunlight is one of the best cures. Let the baby run naked as much as possible. Each time you change the diapers, wash the baby's bottom with water. A little Basic H diluted with 10 parts water can also be used, but be sure to rinse it off. Change the diapers frequently, and be sure to change them right after each bowel movement as the feces irritate the skin.

If the rash is persistent, despite all the procedures recommended above, and all the remedies recommended below, have the baby's urine tested by a medical worker or do it yourself with Squibb's nitrazine papers or some other device available in drugstores. If the urine is too alkaline, then the mother (if the child is nursing) and/or child should eat an alkaline diet. This will cause the child's urine to have an acidic reaction and may help to eliminate the rash.

Acid and alkaline are confusing terms to use in the context of diet, because in this context we call foods such as citrus fruits alkaline. In fact, this does not refer to the acid content of the food but rather to a process that occurs within the body. Foods combine with oxygen and then are "burned up" by the body, thus leaving a residue or "ash." This residue is then analyzed for its mineral content. If it is highest in sodium, potassium, calcium, and magnesium, it is called alkaline producing. If it is highest in sulfur, phosphorus, chlorine, and uncombusted organic acid radicals, it is called acid producing. Try the following diet for two weeks. If you like the results, you may want to continue it longer.

More than two-thirds of your diet should be alkaline-forming foods. This includes almost all vegetables and fruits. (The exceptions are cranberries and large plums or prunes, which have a slightly acid reaction.) All vegetables, including potatoes and sweet potatoes are alkaline. Also lima beans, dried peas, red beans, soybeans (including soy sauce, miso, tofu, etc.), almonds, chestnuts, honey, sunflower seed oil, and sesame seed oil are alkaline.

The following foods are neutral or nearly neutral and can be eaten freely: blueberries, apples, watermelon, sweet corn, fresh green peas, asparagus, olive oil, filbert nuts, egg yolks, butter, goat's milk, cheese, nonfat raw milk (whole milk is more acidic), and chocolate.

Less than one-third of your diet should be selected from acid-forming foods, such as grains, beans (except those listed above) and lentils, nuts (except those listed above), meat, fish, poultry, sugar, and egg whites.

A sample diet might go as follows. For breakfast: cornmeal mush with milk, or fruit with yogurt, or a vegetable omelet with one piece of toast and butter. Snack: apple. Lunch: vegetable soup with a roll, or a large salad with an open-faced grilled cheese sandwich with mushrooms and alfalfa sprouts. Snack: celery sticks with peanut butter. Dinner: stir-fried rice with vegetables, or baked potato with broccoli and fish or meat, or refried red beans with tortillas and lettuce and tomato and a sprinkling of grated cheese. For beverages, drink 1 glass each of apple juice, carrot juice, and milk.

The following remedies will soothe dry, chapped, or "burned" skin.

If the diaper rash is very persistent, and none of the remedies is effective, see your pediatrician. Your baby may have a yeast infection or some other problem that requires medication.

Wheat Germ Oil or Vitamin E Oil. Both oils are soothing and promote rapid healing. Vitamin E oil is squeezed out of a capsule; use a pin to puncture the ends. Apply as needed.

A & D Ointment. This is also used with good results.

Calendula Ointment. Calendula ointment is an excellent homeopathic salve for diaper burn. This ointment is available at some health food and herb stores, and wherever naturopathic and homeopathic remedies are sold (see Resources).

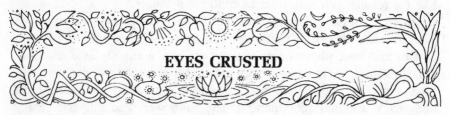

EYES CRUSTED

With some babies, the tear duct at the inner corner of the eye, which drains into the nose, isn't fully developed. Consequently, during the first 3 to 4 weeks of life—or later—the baby may wake up with its eyes crusted shut. This is nothing to worry about, and usually passes by itself. Have a doctor check to make sure it isn't more serious. The doctor may show you how to do a simple massage along the side of the baby's nose to encourage drainage of the duct. The crust can be cleaned off with a cotton ball dipped in one of the eye rinses described in the section on Eyes in chapter 2.

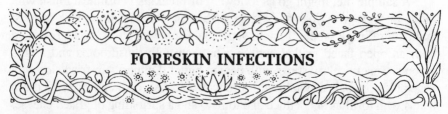

FORESKIN INFECTIONS

At around 2 years of age, a boy's urine tends to become concentrated and irritating. He should drink a lot of water, which dilutes the urine. If the foreskin becomes swollen, painful, or oozy, the following treatments can be used.

Cornstarch Soak. Dilute 1 tablespoon of cornstarch in 1/4 cup warm water. Soak a small clean cloth in this solution, then hold it up to the foreskin for a minute or two. Repeat this 3 times a day. The swelling should go down the first day and should go away entirely in a day or two.

Cider Vinegar. Dilute 1/2 teaspoon of apple cider vinegar in 1/4 cup warm water and apply as with the cornstarch soak above.

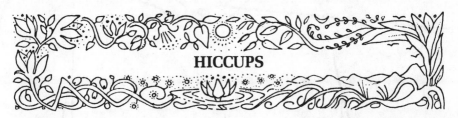

HICCUPS

Hiccups occur to the young and old, but for some reason, children have more than a fair share of them. This is one place where the traditional old-time remedies have held their own. Everyone has their favorite remedies, and here's mine.

Lie Down and Drink Water. Like holding the breath, this one probably works by taking the mind off the problem. Children can use this method from the time they are about 5 years old. Fill a glass or cup half-full with water and have the child lie on his or her back on the floor without a pillow. If necessary, the child can tilt his or her head forward a little. Then have the child slowly drink all the water. By the time the water is gone, the hiccups should be gone also.

Pressure Massage. This one doesn't work immediately, but the hiccups usually go away within a minute or two. I've known hiccups to last for hours, but after this massage, they stop.

The 4 points are located in relation to the sternum (the breast bone) as illustrated. Apply pressure to each point for about 10 seconds. The pressure should be firm, but not painful.

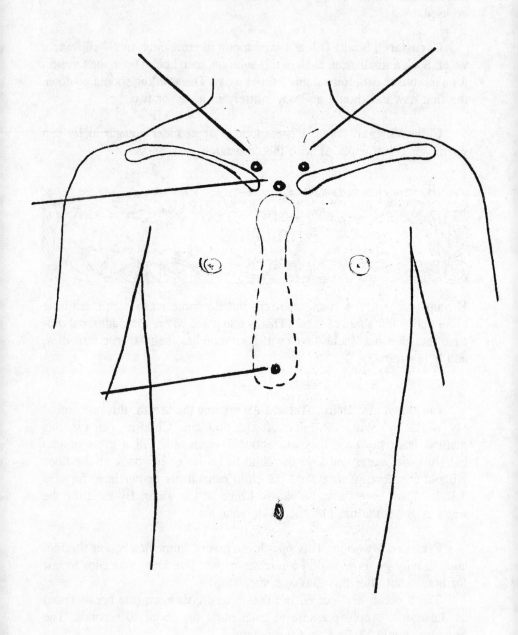

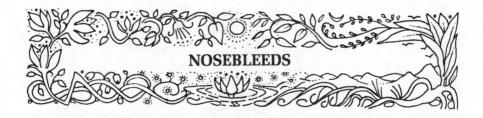

NOSEBLEEDS

An occasional nosebleed is fairly common among children. Since the nose is prominently at the center of the face, it represents self-image. A child who suffers from frequent nosebleeds needs to be noticed.

There are many ways to deal with nosebleeds, and everyone swears by their own method. Nosebleeds aren't very serious, and it isn't hard to stop one. Try to be calm and matter-of-fact so as not to scare the child. Applying pressure is a first-aid method that should take care of the occasional nosebleed.

Applying Pressure. Have the child sit in a straight-back chair with the head straight, in a normal position, or slightly forward if that's more comfortable. Avoid putting the head back, because that makes the child swallow blood. Immediately put a tissue to the nose to soak up the blood and have the child squeeze his or her nose shut, firmly but gently, and hold it that way while breathing through the mouth. If the child is quite young, you can do this for them, while explaining what you are doing. Pressure is a simple first-aid method to stop bleeding. After applying pressure for about 5 minutes, release the nose very slowly to see if the bleeding continues. If it does, insert a small amount of tissue paper or cotton into the nostril. Then squeeze the nose gently. This aids in clotting.

Acupressure for Children. See the section on middle ear infections in chapter 2 (see Index) for a description of acupressure techniques.

Press gently at the B12 point shown on the illustration and described below. Do this twice in 1 week. Most children stop having nosebleeds altogether, or else they experience only mild, occasional attacks.

B12 is located in the back of the head, on the natural hairline, on the side toward the ear of the large muscle that runs down the back of the neck. Anatomically, it is just below the base of the occiput, between the transverse process of the first and second cervical vertebrae, on the lateral border of the insertion of the trapezius. This is known as Bladder 12, T'ien Chu.

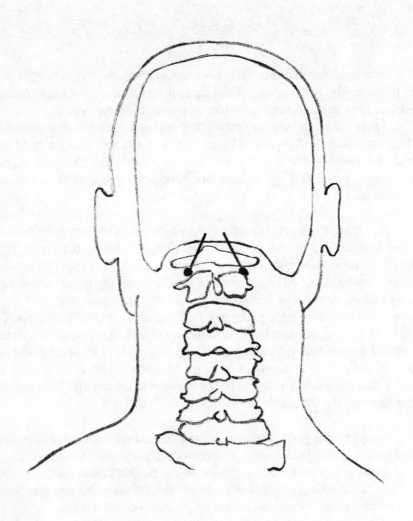

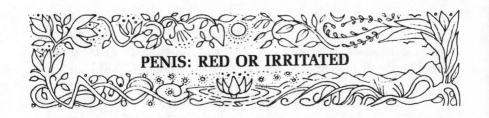

PENIS: RED OR IRRITATED

Calendula Cerate. This homeopathic salve is made of pot marigold flowers. Just apply as needed. This ointment is available at some health food and herb stores, and wherever naturopathic and homeopathic remedies are sold (see Resources).

Aloe Vera. The gel can be used directly from the plant. Break off a small piece of leaf, slit the leaf sideways to expose the gel, and apply as needed. The fresh gel from the plant is more effective than the bottled gel, which is available in some health food stores.

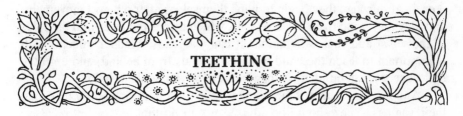

TEETHING

The following remedies can be used to relieve the pain of teething.

Clove Powder. This is applied to the gums to act as a mild, local anesthetic. Mix 1/4 teaspoon of clove powder with a few drops of water to make a paste. Apply to the gums around the area where the tooth is coming through. If the cloves seem to disturb the child, remove the paste after a minute or two. You might want to try it yourself, so you'll know how it feels.

Alcohol. The most popular, time-honored remedy for teething babies (and their poor parents) is booze. A good method is to soak a gauze pad in brandy and apply to the gums. Or just dip your finger in some form of drinking alcohol and rub the gums. It's best to avoid giving the child alcohol to drink since not all infants can tolerate alcohol.

Vitamin C. Teething often can be relieved by giving 500 to 1000 mg. of vitamin C 1 to 3 times a day while the child is in pain. Ascorbic acid crystals dissolve easily in water or juice and can be taken by the dropper or in a bottle. If the child is sick or feverish, vitamin C will help.

Hylands Teething Tablets. This is a homeopathic remedy. Each tablet contains lime phosphate, chamomilla, coffea, and belladonna. Instructions are given on the bottle. The tablets are available in some health food stores, and can be ordered from the Standard Homeopathic Company (see Resources).

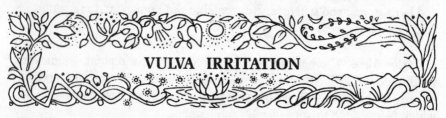

VULVA IRRITATION

The vulva sometimes gets irritated when little girls are around the age of 3 or 4. At this age, they begin to wipe themselves after a bowel movement, and they may wipe from back to front, which brings the feces into the folds of the vulva and causes irritation. It can also cause bladder infections. It is important to teach the child to wipe the anus from behind, and until the child becomes good at it, it may be best for an adult to help.

Another cause of irritation is that little girls put things (like dirt) into their vaginas. They should be advised not to do this.

Irritation of the vulva can also be caused by wearing nylon tights or other clothing that keeps moisture in.

Bubble baths are another offender, and some soaps are also irritating. Basic H is a soap with a pH of 6.5, similar to normal human skin. It can be diluted in 5 to 10 parts water before using as a soap. Or 1 to 2 teaspoons can be added to a bath to make a healthy bubble bath. Basic H is available from Shaklee distributors (consult the Yellow Pages under Health Foods).

Calendula Tincture. Dilute one part tincture with 10 parts water and apply with cotton to the vulva, being sure to get into all the folds. Do this 3 or more times a day.

Yogurt. Apply plain yogurt to the vagina 3 times a day.

Chapter 4

Eliminating Toxins

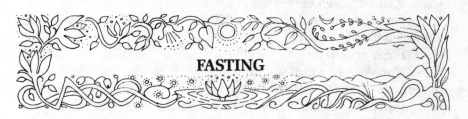

FASTING

The digestive system is constantly at work, processing every crazy thing we deliver to it. It's healthful to give this system a rest now and then.

Fasting is not for everyone. It certainly isn't for diabetics, or hypoglycemics, or people who have active tuberculosis or a weak heart, or who have to take strong drugs every day (such as cortisone, digitalis, or chemotherapy). Since you don't want to put toxins into the system while trying to clean them out, it doesn't work to smoke or drink coffee, alcohol, or soft drinks while you are fasting.

Fasting should not be a form of self-torture. If you are not accustomed to abstaining from food, then do it gradually.

The One-Third Rule

This plan makes fasting easier to stay with.

1. Decide how long you are going to fast (begin with 1 day).

2. Allow one-third of that time to prepare for your fast and one-third of that time to come off the fast. For example, if you want to fast for 1 day (3 meals), begin by having a simple dinner the night before (avoid concentrated proteins such as beans, milk, cheese, and meat). Fast for 1 full day. Then have a simple breakfast the next day (for example, fruit with yogurt or cooked cereal, instead of eggs or bacon). Avoid all refined and processed foods, including sugar. This helps your digestive system adjust to your fast.

3. After breaking a fast, be careful not to overeat, and chew your food thoroughly. If you break your fast slowly, you'll enhance your appreciation of foods, improve your self-control, and diminish your desire for unhealthy foods.

Various Fasts

Decide what kind of fast you want. Here are some choices.

1. Total fast, with only water.

2. Fast with blood-cleansing herbal teas (see the section later in this chapter on blood-cleansing).

3. Fresh juice fast.

4. Mono diet in which you drink liquids (herb teas, fresh juices) and eat only one of the following foods, but as much as you like. A good quality plain yogurt can be chosen, and a little raw honey, molasses, or maple syrup can be added for extra energy, if needed. Or you can fast with just one fruit per meal or preferably one fruit per day, up to about 2 pounds. Any fruit can be used, but grapes, papayas, grapefruit, apples, and watermelons are particularly cleansing. A vegetable fast means eating just one vegetable per meal or preferably one vegetable per day, up to 2 pounds. Any vegetable can be used, but carrots are nutritious and filling. With a grain fast you eat just one grain per meal or preferably one grain per day. Brown rice is a favorite, and usually condiments are allowed also, such as salt, tamari (soy sauce), and gomasio (roasted ground sesame seeds with a little salt). Be sure to chew thoroughly.

A mono diet is easier than a regular fast, especially if you experience hunger pangs or weakness while fasting. It can also be used as an introduction to a long fast, by preceding a regular fast with a day or two of mono-fasting. A mono diet is helpful to the body, because it puts limited demands on the digestive system.

Eliminating Protein

If you are fasting to rid the body of disease, then fast with fruits or vegetables or preferably just liquids. It's important to temporarily withdraw protein, which forces the body to "consume" itself. After 3 days, your body will live on its own substance. It will digest its own tissues. The first cells to be digested are the ones that are diseased, damaged, aged, or dead. Enzymes can chemically change or dissolve apparently hard growths. Thus, cholesterol can be removed and tumors, abscesses, and cysts will literally melt away. Even enlarged joints can be reduced. These diseased cells act as protein for the body, providing the amino acids necessary for building new cells.

How Long to Fast

For general health and weight control, fast 1 day a week, and then once a month for 3 days. For minor problems, a 1-day to 3-day fast is often helpful. For more serious problems, a 7-day to 10-day fast is recommended. Therapeutic fasts for severe illnesses usually last for 2 to 4 weeks and are repeated 2, 6, or 12 months later. After the age of 30, a fast of 3 to 10 days is recommended once a year to rejuvenate the body and increase the life span. After the age of 45, this should be increased to twice a year.

Do not undertake a fast longer than 10 days without supervision from a naturopathic doctor, a nutritionist, or a person skilled in supervising fasts.

I know of several cases where prolonged fasting caused malnutrition or an intolerance to food. (In such cases, a baked potato without the skin and without condiments can be used to ease a person back into a tolerance for food.)

During a long fast, most people are surprised to discover that after the first day, their hunger pangs actually diminish; by the third day, they rarely experience any hunger at all. Most people describe a remarkable sense of well-being and good energy. Some people find they are able to carry on their normal activities. Others prefer to retreat into the woods or mountains, and to use the inner calmness they feel for introspection, rest, and meditation.

But people who undertake long fasts often don't know when to stop fasting. A normally healthy male living under peaceful circumstances could go for 90 to 100 days without food. But an emaciated and sickly person reaches the danger zone sooner.

I urge people who are embarking on a long fast to remember to end their fast when they begin to feel hungry. Eventually—and usually within 28 days—the hunger pangs return, and this is the best time to begin slowly breaking your fast. But even if you feel no hunger after 28 days, it's still advisable to break your fast and consider doing another one after you've allowed your body at least 2 months to stabilize.

Hunger pains are not to be confused with a healing crisis.

The Healing Crisis

If you are trying to get rid of a disease and your body is full of toxins, waste material is being thrown into the bloodstream so rapidly that the organs of elimination can't handle it all. You may experience unpleasant headaches, skin eruptions, fever, swollen joints, pain, and temporary worsening of your condition. This is not the time to quit; take it as a good sign. The healing crisis should pass in a day or two, and then you'll notice a significant improvement in your condition.

However, you can eliminate the discomfort by helping the elimination process. The best way to do this is with a coffee enema, which is discussed later in this chapter.

Guidelines for Fasting

An excellent book on fasting is *How to Keep Slim, Healthy and Young With Juice Fasting* by Paavo O. Airola (Health Publishers, P.O. Box 22001, Phoenix, Arizona 85028). There is also an extensive section on fasting in Airola's book, *How To Get Well*, which is available in most health food stores and bookstores.

Sweeteners. These are usually discouraged, but if there's a significant loss of energy or faintness or a strong craving for sweets, I allow a teaspoon of raw honey or molasses or maple syrup, because it's easily assimilated and boosts the blood sugar and gives energy. For such people, a mono diet will generally be more tolerable.

Vitamins. These are not usually taken, particularly the oil soluble vitamins (A, D, E, and K), which need to be taken with oil-containing foods in order to be properly digested.

Exercise. Fresh air, sunlight, and exercise are highly recommended.

Bathing. A daily hot bath followed by a cold bath is excellent for the circulation. Precede the bath by rubbing the whole body with a skin brush, or use a loofa sponge during the bath. One-third of all body impurities and wastes are eliminated through the skin.

Enemas. The toxic wastes built up by fasting would ordinarily be eliminated with the feces, but during fasting the bowel movements cease, and the toxins remain in the colon and get reabsorbed, poisoning the system and putting a strain on the liver and kidneys. An enema cleanses the system. It should be taken each morning or each night. If you have a severe condition, take 2 enemas per day.

The Short Fast

There are many ways to fast, but this is one of the most popular.

First Third. As explained under the One-Third Rule earlier, during the first third of the fast, eat only fruits, vegetables, and grains. Avoid concentrated proteins such as meat, dairy, and beans. Avoid sugars and refined foods.

Fasting Days. You may drink plain water or fresh fruit juice or fresh vegetable juice. You may wish to dilute it with up to 50 percent water. Sip the juice slowly, mixing it well with saliva. Use a laxative at end of the day, or take an enema once a day.

Last Third. Follow the same guidelines as for the first third. It is *extremely important* to break a fast slowly, or else you can develop a lot of gas and abdominal discomfort.

The Long Fast

As explained above, most people can fast safely for up to 28 days. The body will begin by consuming unnecessary fat, and will end up consuming diseased tissue. An obese person, therefore, can fast much longer than an emaciated person. This should be taken into consideration when deciding whether to fast for 2, 3, or 4 weeks.

When fasting for longer than 1 week, it's advisable to have the supervision of a medical person. Ask this person to take your blood pressure every few days. If the diastolic is below 60, or the systolic is below 90, it is advisable to bring your fast to an end (slowly). The medical person should also observe the tone of your flesh and watch for any atrophy of the muscles and sloppiness instead of firmness of flesh.

Following a therapeutic fast, it's most effective to maintain—at least for a couple of weeks—a good diet that is very low in concentrated proteins. The macrobiotic diet or a raw foods diet have been used effectively.

Juice Fasting

In a normal adult, about half the body cells are mature and functioning at optimum level, while one-fourth are maturing, and another one-fourth are aging and dying. When these dead and dying cells are eliminated quickly, the production of new cells is stimulated.

Juice is like predigested food. The juicer eliminates everything that is not digestible. The juices provide vitamins, minerals, enzymes, and trace elements without the additional burden of bulk. The generous amount of minerals in juices helps restore the biochemical and mineral balance in the tissues and cells. Meanwhile, the liver and kidneys are relieved of their usual role in the digestion of food, and can turn instead to the quick and efficient elimination of wastes and toxins from the body.

Fasting on fresh raw fruit and vegetable juices, vegetable broths, and herbal teas causes much faster recovery from disease, and more effective cleansing and rejuvenation of the tissues than a plain water fast.

Fruit and vegetable juices are alkaline and help eliminate uric acids and other inorganic acids. The natural sugars in fresh juice strengthen the heart.

The most nutritious form of juice fasting is to prepare fresh juices and drink them immediately. There are various kinds of juicers, but a favorite is the Champion. This is a masticating juicer, as opposed to the centrifugal type.

A centrifugal juicer grates the vegetables and then extracts the juice by high speed thrust. A masticating juicer rubs, "chews," and breaks up the cells and fibers of the vegetables and then forces the juice from the vegetables under pressure. This method extracts a greater amount of enzymes, trace minerals, and vitamins from the cells and fibers.

The Champion is also very convenient because it eliminates the pulp as it works, so you don't have to stop and clean it as often.

An excellent juice for fasting is carrot and beet juice. Use only one-fourth or less of beets, because they're very strong. They will stimulate the gall bladder to release bile, which encourages elimination. But be forewarned it will turn your stools red.

For those who don't have a juicer, a grape juice fast can be very effective, as described in *Grape Cure*, a little book by Joanna Brandt.

Lemon juice is another excellent cleanser, and many people like the fast described in Stanley Burrough's *The Master Cleanser*, which uses lemon juice, water, and maple syrup, with laxatives instead of enemas.

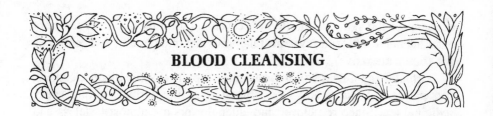

BLOOD CLEANSING

The idea of cleansing the blood of toxins and impurities is basic to herbal medicine. Herbs that can do this are referred to as *alteratives*, and they are believed to improve assimilation by catalyzing mineral salts in the blood; to improve excretion by stimulating the kidneys, liver, and lungs to secrete impurities from the blood and by stimulating and cleansing the lymph glands; and to improve nutrition by strengthening the digestive organs.

The term *tonic* has a similar definition. It refers to the strengthening properties of herbs to stimulate the appetite and improve digestion.

I can't guarantee that any blood cleanser will do all of the above, but I've seen good results with various skin conditions and sinusitis from the use of blood cleansers, combined with fasting and/or simplifying the diet. Many schools of medicine agree that skin eruptions (acne, eczema, psoriasis, herpes) are the body's way of getting rid of toxins that have accumulated in the body and which cannot escape through the usual channels (urine, feces, sweat). Constipation is one cause of this condition, and if this is a problem, be sure to treat it also. But underactive organs of elimination are another cause (liver, kidneys, lungs, lymph glands, and skin). Other conditions which sometimes respond well to blood-cleansers are bladder infections, menstrual difficulties, and menopause.

The most common and well-known blood-cleansers are the red foods: beets, cherries, blackberries, grapes, red cabbage, and cranberries. Cranberry juice is an excellent blood-cleanser. The juice you purchase at grocery store will work, but many people prefer to avoid the added sugar. Some health food stores carry a cranberry juice concentrate that does not have sugar. Drink at least 1/2 cup of juice 3 times a day for 1 week. During the second week, drink at least 1/2 cup twice a day. During the third week, drink at least 1/2 cup once a day. It's harmless, so if you feel like drinking more than this amount, just follow your instincts.

There are many herbal blood-cleansers, but these are my favorites: red clover (alterative), elder flowers (alterative), burdock root (alterative and excellent for the skin), nettle (tonic), cayenne (hot tonic), golden seal root (bitter alterative and tonic), yarrow (alterative and bitter tonic), and echinacea root (bitter alterative).

Virtually any illness will improve more rapidly if some blood-cleansing takes place, so I like to add 1 or 2 blood-cleansing herbs to almost every medicinal tea. Since red clover and elder flowers are almost tasteless and grow in great abundance in most locations, these are the herbs I usually choose. I also like nettle, because it's quite palatable and very high in minerals. If there's a skin condition, then burdock is essential.

The following tea combines the properties of several blood-cleansing herbs with peppermint, which has a pleasant flavor and a beneficial effect on the stomach, nerves, and circulation.

Recipe: Blood Cleansing Tea. Bring 6 cups of water to a boil, then add 2 teaspoons burdock root and 2 teaspoons echinacea root. Simmer for 10 minutes, then add 2 teaspoons nettle. Simmer for 10 more minutes, remove from the heat, then add 2 teaspoons red clover, 2 teaspoons elder flowers, and 2 teaspoons peppermint. Brew in a covered container for 5 minutes. Then strain. Add honey if desired, Drink in the same quantities as indicated for cranberry juice, above.

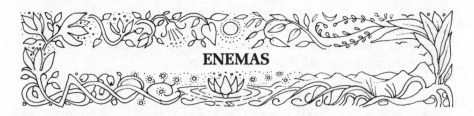

ENEMAS

Most of the old herbalists and many of the modern ones are staunch advocates of enemas as a part of healing any serious illness. Illness is understood as a toxic process, and proper cleansing of the body is considered vital before nourishment with herbs or diet can make a lasting difference.

Cleansing the body refers not only to the body's plumbing (the gastrointestinal tract consisting of the esophagus, stomach, small intestines, large intestines, and anus) but also the organs that remove toxins from the body (the liver, kidneys, lungs, lymph glands, and skin).

Coffee Enemas

When caffeine is taken through the rectum, it has been observed in animals that the bile ducts open and more bile flows. When the coffee is retained for 15 minutes, the caffeine is absorbed through the hemorrhoidal veins and into the liver. The increased flow of bile stimulates the liver to dump its accumulation of poison, which is carried out with the feces. This then causes the liver to function more effectively.

Ironically, this therapy is used when drinking coffee is strictly forbidden. For example, one woman had a cyst in her breast, which is known to be aggravated by caffeine. She found that even a half cup of coffee would increase the tenderness of the cyst. Yet the cyst disappeared within a week just by drinking fresh carrot and beet juice and by taking coffee enemas daily. Whenever she took a coffee enema, the tenderness in her breast actually *decreased* within 10 to 15 minutes.

Here's how to give yourself a coffee enema:

1. You must be right next to the toilet, so do whatever is necessary to make your bathroom floor comfortable. You can fold a washable blanket (you probably won't need to wash it) in 3 or 4 sections, as a padding, and put it on the floor. Cover this with a towel (you may have to wash this because there might be some spill from the coffee). Have another towel to cover yourself. Put down a pillow. Get a book or something light that you might enjoy reading. If it's cool, set up a heater. Put a hook on the wall near where you'll be lying, at 2 to 3 feet above the floor, to hang the enema bag. You'll also need a watch or a clock. You may enjoy some relaxing music.

2. You'll need a 1-quart enema bag. This can be purchased in any drugstore. They usually come with 2 nozzles and can be used interchangeably as a douche or enema bag. The long nozzle with many holes is for douching. The short nozzle with 1 hole is for enemas.

3. Bring 3 cups of water to a boil and add 3 heaping tablespoons of drip grind (not instant) coffee. Boil for 3 minutes, then simmer for 15 minutes. Strain. Add 1 cup or more of cool water so you have a total of 1 quart of warm coffee. Make sure the clamp of the enema bag is within about 10 inches of the nozzle. Close the clamp. Pour the coffee into the bag. Put the nozzle in the sink or tub and release the clamp for a moment to let out a little coffee. This releases the air from the hose. Clamp the hose again and hang the bag from the hook.

4. First, use the toilet. Then undress from the waist down. Lie on the towel on your right side (the liver is on the right side, and this helps the caffeine get to the liver), with your knees drawn up toward your chest in a comfortable fetal position. Then insert the nozzle into your anus. If this is difficult, then bear down as if you were having a bowel movement, because this causes the anus to open. If necessary, apply a little oil or salve to the nozzle. When the nozzle has been inserted, cover yourself if you feel chilly. Inhale to the count of 7, and exhale to the count of 7. Continue doing this until your breath is deep and steady. Then contract your anus (as if you were restraining the urge to defecate), and reach back and *slowly* release the clamp (you may want to hold the clamp only half open so the coffee enters very slowly). Continue breathing steadily and deeply. Allow the coffee to flow in slowly. When it feels like you've got as much as you can hold, clamp the hose. You can relax your anus while you rest. Wait as long as necessary until you feel you might be able to take some more. Continue breathing deeply. When and if you feel ready, repeat this process, until the whole bag has been emptied or until you are holding as much as you can hold. (If you have difficulty holding a full quart, in the future you may want to do a quick plain water enema and release it before doing the coffee enema.)

Now breathe deeply and concentrate on relaxing for 15 minutes. You may be able to read. At times you may feel a strong desire to release the enema, but this can usually be resisted by deep breathing or by short, shallow panting. The urge should pass within a minute.

5. When the 15 minutes are completed, close the clamp and remove the nozzle (be prepared for a bit of coffee to come out of the nozzle), and get onto the toilet. There will probably be a quick expulsion from the bowel. Stay on the toilet, at least 5 minutes, breathing deeply, and kneading your abdomen to help release the enema completely. When you feel finished, you can get up, but you may feel a quick urge to use the bathroom again one or more times within the next hour or so.

6. You may find after an enema that you feel exhilarated. Colors may appear brighter, and your senses may be more attuned. Be aware of what you put into your body at this time: Avoid sugar, dairy products (except for plain yogurt or kefir), meat, and drugs of any kind for about 24 hours. A fresh juice fast is well-suited to combine with an enema.

Note: During and shortly after an enema, people tend to feel extremely vulnerable. It's a good time to lie quietly and allow yourself to get in touch with your feelings. The gastro-intestinal tract is the seat of the emotions, and invading it is like "stirring up a nest of worms." Indeed, if the body is harboring worms, they will be washed out by this process. Allow your emotions to come to the surface. Express them in any way you can. You may want to seek counseling, because clearing up these emotions may be an essential part of healing your disease.

For some people coffee enemas are too stimulating. Then it is better to use herbs that are good for the liver. Vegetarians and non-coffee drinkers, as well as people whose bodies are very sensitive, may find that coffee enemas sometimes make them jittery, or cause gas, and cause some tenderness in the liver.

Use coffee enemas for extreme cleansing, for very severe illnesses and severe pain, but once you have improved, try a dandelion root enema (see below). For example, with a 3-day fast, try a coffee enema on the first day, dandelion root on the second day, and water on the third day. The effect of such a program is so cleansing that anyone who is over 30 years old, and anyone who is ill, would do well to follow it once a month, indefinitely. After the age of 30, the system tends to become sluggish. A good monthly cleansing is a tool for a long and healthy life. Most of us do at least a monthly cleansing of our homes!

Dandelion Root Enema. Bring 1 quart of water to a boil. Add 4 teaspoons dandelion root and simmer for 20 minutes. Strain, and use as directed under coffee enema, above.

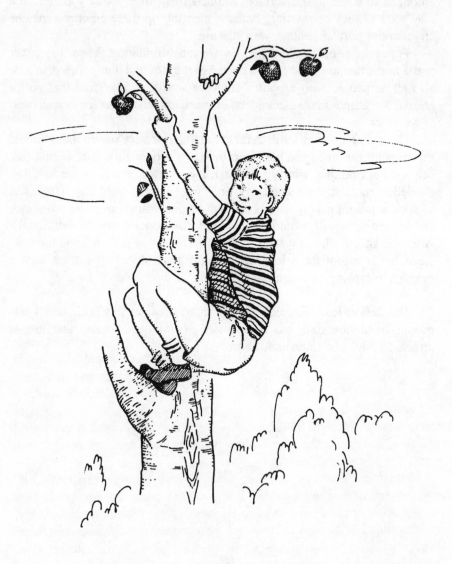

Chapter 5

Vitamins and Minerals

The Minimum Daily Requirements (MDR) given here are for perfectly healthy people living without stress, in a healthy environment. Since this does not describe most people, it is up to you to adjust your intake as needed.

VITAMIN A

Minimum Daily Requirements: Lactating Women: 8000 I.U.
Pregnant Women: 6000 I.U.
Men, Women, Boys, Girls: 5000 I.U.
Children under 11: 2500 I.U.

Vitamin A, a fat-soluble vitamin, builds resistance to infections, especially of the respiratory tract. It permits the formation of visual purple in the eye, counteracting night blindness, weak eyesight, and light sensitivity. Vitamin A also promotes healthy skin. It is essential for pregnancy and lactation, and it increases longevity and delays senility. A lack of vitamin A causes night blindness; light sensitivity; increased susceptibility to infections; dry, scaly, or oily skin; defective teeth with a thin and weak enamel; and retarded growth.

Symptoms of excess have been seen in people taking over 100,000 I.U. per day for over a year. Adelle Davis claims that even with such high dosage, toxicity can be prevented by taking adequate vitamin C (presumably, at least 100 mg. a day). Symptoms of overdose are thinning hair, sore lips, bruising, nosebleeds, headaches, blurred vision, flaking, itching skin, painful joints, and tenderness and swelling over the long bones. Lab experiments with animals have shown that vitamin A overdose during a critical period in pregnancy is one of the factors in the development of cleft palate. The same symptom can result when a mother's diet is deficient in this vitamin.

For best absorption of vitamin A, vitamin E is necessary. Fat is also required, so if you take this or any other fat-soluble vitamin between meals, it's advisable to wash them down with whole milk. Bile is another requirement, so if there's a disease or removal of the gall bladder, take supplementary bile tablets and lecithin when taking this vitamin.

Note: Antacid pills, when taken in excess, neutralize the hydrochloric acid in the stomach, making it difficult to break down fats, including the fat-soluble vitamins. This impairs absorption of vitamins A, D, and K. Mineral oil (including vaseline, baby oil, and many cosmetic oils) is absorbed through the skin and taken into the body, where it traps your fat-soluble vitamins, which are then excreted along with the oil. Olive and other vegetable oils can be substituted. Fluorescent lighting can cause your need for vitamin A to increase rapidly after prolonged exposure. Contact lenses can also increase your need for this vitamin. During illness, the need for vitamin A is increased because absorption is poor and the storage of vitamin A in the liver is impaired.

Foods Highest in Vitamin A (over 5000 I.U.). Fish liver oil, liver, beet greens, broccoli, carrots, cauliflower, swiss chard, collard greens, dandelion greens, endive, kale, lamb's quarters, loose leaf lettuce, mustard greens, spinach, winter squash, sweet potatoes, tomatoes, turnip greens, watercress, apricots, cantaloupe, cherries, papayas, peaches, prunes.

B COMPLEX

The water-soluble B vitamins work as a team. If you get an excess of one B vitamin, your body will excrete the ones that are deficient. (Niacin, B3, is the one B vitamin that can be taken alone without throwing the others off balance.) Unfortunately, folic acid and PABA (members of the B family) are regulated by the Food and Drug Administration, and the amounts allowed are so small that it unbalances the proportions of the other B vitamins. Folic acid is regulated because it masks pernicious anemia (which is usually caused by a vitamin B12 deficiency). This could be remedied by including B12 in B complex supplements that contain folic acid (which is usually done anyway). PABA is regulated because it is a sulfa drug suppressant. This regulation dates back to the days when the use of sulfa drugs were widespread.

The best way to get the whole B complex is with plenty of B vitamins in your diet, and by encouraging the manufacture of this vitamin in your intestines. To do this, eat at least 1 tablespoon of yogurt and drink 1/4 cup of milk daily (or eat 1/4 cup of yogurt). The yogurt encourages the growth of intestinal lactobacilli and the milk gives them a medium to grow on. Since they also thrive on roughage, eat plenty of vegetables. One of the best nonmeat sources of B vitamins is whole grains. Try to avoid refined foods. Also avoid coffee, alcohol, and diuretics, which wash out your B vitamins. The best food supplements are torula or brewer's yeast (about 1 tablespoon per day), liver (preferably organic, once a week), and wheat germ (try to get it fresh).

If tablets are taken, get the whole B complex in a supplement that contains equal amounts of B2 and B6. Take before or after eating, because they should combine with food for maximum effectiveness.

B1 (Thiamine)

Minimum Daily Requirement: Lactating Women, Men, Boys: 1.2 mg.
Pregnant Women, Girls: 1 mg.
Women: .8 mg.
Children under 11: .6 mg.

Vitamin B1 is essential for the breakdown of carbohydrates into glucose, which is then oxidized by the body to produce energy. It is also essential for normal functioning of nerve tissues, muscles, and the heart. A lack of vitamin B1 may lead to a loss of appetite, weakness and lassitude, nervous irritability, insomnia, loss of weight, vague aches and pains, mental depression, and constipation. In children, it may impair growth. In severe cases of deficiency, beriberi may result. Since B1 is essential for a healthy nervous system, a lack of it will manifest as a loss of ankle and knee jerk reflexes, neuritis, or muscular weakness in the feet, calves, and thighs. Psychological symptoms of deficiency include mental instability, poor memory, vague fears, uneasiness, and ideas of persecution.

Foods Highest in Vitamin B1 (over 5 mg.). These include brewer's or torula yeast (1 teaspoon), pork, organ meats, soy flour, brown rice, whole wheat flour (1 cup each), wheat germ (1/3 cup), Brazil nuts (1/2 cup), natural peanut butter (1/3 cup), and sunflower seeds (3 tablespoon).

B2

Minimum Daily Requirements: Lactating Women, Boys: 1.8 mg.
Men: 1.7 mg.
Girls, Pregnant Women: 1.5 mg.
Women: 1.3 mg.
Children under 11: 1 mg.

Vitamin B2 improves growth and promotes general health. It is essential for healthy eyes, skin, and mouth and important for respiration. A lack of vitamin B2 can result in eyes that itch, burn, become bloodshot, or develop dimness of vision or cataracts. The mouth may become inflamed or develop sores; the tongue may become purplish or inflamed at tip and margin; there may be cracking at corners of lips. There may be a degeneration of nervous tissues, resulting in loss of coordination, mental confusion, and loss of muscular strength in arms and legs.

Foods Highest in Vitamin B2 (over 5 mg.). These include liver, kidney, milk (1 cup), brewer's yeast (2 tablespoons), torula yeast (1 teaspoon), cottage cheese, turnip greens, macaroni and cheese, wheat germ (1 cup), almonds.

B3

Vitamin B3 is also known as niacin. It comes in three synthetic forms: nicotinic acid, niacinamide, and nicotinamide. Nicotinic acid causes a flushing and itching of the face and skin, whereas niacinamide minimizes or eliminates this reaction.

Minimum Daily Requirements: Pregnant Women: 21 mg.
Boys, Lactating Women: 20 mg.
Men: 19 mg.
Girls: 17 mg.
Women: 14 mg.
Children under 11: 11 mg.

Vitamin B3 is important for proper functioning of the nervous system. It promotes growth, maintains normal function of the gastro-intestinal tract, is necessary for metabolism of sugar, and helps to maintain normal skin condition. A lack of vitamin B3 causes a sore tongue, dysfunction of the nervous system, mental depression and irritability. There may be fatigue headaches and vague aches and pains, as well as a loss of appetite and weight, nausea, vomiting, and abdominal pains. Psychological symptoms of deficiency range from loss of memory to stupor or mania.

Pellagra, characterized by the above symptoms and caused by a deficiency mostly of vitamins B3 and B2, begins with an inflamed mouth and red, sore tongue. Then cracks and sores appear in skin and mouth. Dietary deficiency of B3 is usually accompanied by a deficiency of B1, B2, and B6.

Foods Highest in Vitamin B3 (over 2.5 mg.). These include meat, poultry, organ meats, fish (excluding shellfish), mushrooms, dried apricots, dried dates, bran flakes, brown or converted rice, rice polish, wheat germ (1 cup), whole wheat, natural peanut butter (2 tablespoons), sunflower seeds (2 tablespoons), brewer's yeast (1 tablespoon), and torula yeast (1 teaspoon).

B6

Minimum Daily Requirements: 5 to 10 mg.

Vitamin B6 aids in food assimilation and in protein and fat metabolism. It prevents various nervous disorders, skin disorders, and nausea. A lack of vitamin B6 may result in nervousness, insomnia, skin eruptions including eczema, loss of muscle control, vomiting, gas, diarrhea, cancer.

Note: Pregnant women are notoriously deficient in B6. Also, the antibiotic streptomycin appears to destroy B6 or to increase the need for it, causing epileptic-type convulsions in children.

Foods Highest in Vitamin B6. These include meat, fish, wheat germ, egg yolk, cantaloupe, cabbage, milk, yeast, whole grains, organ meats. Magnesium is needed for the proper absorption of the vitamin.

B12

Minimum Daily Requirements: 1 to 3 micrograms (mcg.)

Vitamin B12 helps in the formation and regeneration of red blood cells, thus helping to prevent anemia. It promotes growth and increased appetite in children and acts as a general tonic for adults. A lack of B12 may lead to nutritional and pernicious anemia, tiredness, poor appetite, and growth failure in children. Symptoms of a vitamin B12 deficiency include sore mouth and tongue, menstrual disturbances, nerve disorders: "pins and needles" in hands and feet, neuritis, pain and stiffness in spine, difficulty walking.

Foods Highest in Vitamin B12. These include liver, beef, pork, eggs, milk, cheese, fish, organ meats, yeast, wheat germ, and soy beans. Vitamin B6, vitamin C, and adequate protein are needed for the proper absorption of the vitamin.

Note: Strict vegetarians who do not eat eggs or dairy products (vegans) are in danger of developing a B12 deficiency. But it's difficult to detect this deficiency in a vegetarian because it tends to be masked by a high folic acid content in the blood. So nerve damage can occur before the deficiency is detected. Strict vegetarians are advised to take 1 tablet (50 mcg.) of B12 each week.

VITAMIN C

Minimum Daily Requirements: Lactating and Pregnant Women: 100 mg.
Boys, Girls: 80 mg.
Men, Women: 70 mg.

The minimum daily requirements given above are for people who are not under stress. During stress, harmful substances are formed in the body. Vitamin C can detoxify these substances if enough is supplied, but then it is used up and carried away in the urine, so the need for this vitamin is increased. During an infection, vitamin C is quickly destroyed, so the need for this vitamin rises dramatically, in proportion to the seriousness of the infection. Vitamin C can detoxify toxins and foreign substances, but it is destroyed in the process. For example, each cigarette destroys about 25 mg. of vitamin C.

Vitamin C is necessary for healthy teeth, gums, and bones. It strengthens all connective tissue, promotes wound healing, maintains capillary walls, and helps maintain health and energy. It detoxifies the body, giving protection when potentially harmful drugs or x-rays are given. A lack of vitamin C causes soft and bleeding gums, tooth decay, loss of appetite, muscular weakness, bruising, capillary weakness, anemia, nosebleeds, and hemorrhaging. Vitamin C is water soluble.

Excessive intake of vitamin C can lead to a rash (usually caused by the acetone or binder in ascorbic acid pills), acidity, gas, diarrhea (usually caused by megadoses of this vitamin). *Note*: To prevent side effects when taking large doses of vitamin C, take 150 mg. calcium with each 500 mg. of vitamin C.

Treatment of certain severe diseases, such as herpes, call for massive doses of vitamin C. If the dosage gives you diarrhea, reduce your intake until you find the highest amount that will not give you diarrhea, and then maintain that dosage. When taking large doses, take the cheapest form of vitamin C, which is usually ascorbic acid or calcium ascorbate (which is less acidic) powder or crystals. Take 1/4 teaspoon for about 1000 mg. of vitamin C. This can be dissolved in a liquid.

Pantothenic acid (a member of the B complex family) and vitamin B6 are needed for the best absorption of vitamin C.

Foods Highest in Vitamin C (over 25 mg.). The following steamed vegetables are high in vitamin C: beet greens, broccoli, brussel sprouts, cabbage (steamed or raw), cauliflower, collards, dandelion greens, kale, lamb's quarters, mustard greens, spinach, turnip greens, and turnips. Raw kohlrabi, green peppers, tomatoes, watercress, cantaloupe, papaya, rose hips, acerola cherries, and citrus fruits are also high in vitamin C, as is liver.

VITAMIN D

Minimum Daily Requirement: 400 I.U.

The need for this vitamin increases for adolescent girls, people with porous bones (most elderly people), and during illness or stress.

Fat-soluble vitamin D regulates the use of calcium and phosphorus in the body and is therefore necessary for the proper formation of bones and teeth. It is essential for preventing rickets (softening of the bones in children, resulting in bow-legs and other mis-shapen bones). It is important for growth, vigor, and development during infancy and childhood. A lack of vitamin D may lead to various skeletal deformities, such as bow-legs, knock-knees, enlargement of the ends of the long bones, curvature of the spine, softening of the skull, and delayed closing of the anterior fontanel in infants. It may result in retarded growth, lack of vigor, muscular weakness, enlarged parathyroid glands, and tooth decay. A deficiency in vitamin D is associated with low serum calcium and low body phosphorus.

Rickets are no longer common in North America because of vitamin D enriched milk. But dark-skinned people tend to be more vulnerable to it, since the pigment in dark skin blocks absorption of the sun's rays. If a dark-skinned person is also allergic to milk, the problem becomes more serious, especially if the person is living in a place where there is little sunlight. Such a person should take vitamin A, vitamin D, and calcium supplements.

Excessive intake of vitamin D may result in weakness, vomiting, diarrhea, headaches, demineralization of bones, and calcification of soft tissue. There may be muscle spasms, inflammation of the pancreas, convulsions, a kind of diabetes, hypertension, irreversible kidney damage, and even death—with 100,000 to 500,000 units taken daily. With infants, 1800 units can inhibit growth. If taken during pregnancy, the infants may be born with badly shaped jaws with a faulty bite, show signs of mental deficiencies, or suffer obstruction of blood flow. Vitamin D toxicity can be prevented by taking adequate amounts of vitamins C, A, and choline.

Vitamin D is formed in the oil on the skin by summer sunshine. This oil washes off easily, even with cold water, so tanning after swimming or bathing will not produce much vitamin D (though use of suntan oil would probably be just as good. Winter sun produces no vitamin D.

For best absorption of vitamin D, vitamin E is necessary. Fat is also required, so if you take this or any other fat-soluble vitamin between meals, it's advisable to wash them down with whole milk. Bile is another requirement, so if there's a disease or removal of the gall bladder, take supplementary bile tablets and lecithin when taking this vitamin.

Note: Antacid pills, when taken in excess, neutralize the hydrochloric acid in the stomach, making it difficult to break down fats, including the fat-soluble vitamins. This impairs absorption of vitamins A, D, and K. Mineral oil (including vaseline, baby oil, and many cosmetic oils) is absorbed through the skin and taken into the body, where it traps fat-soluble vitamins, which are then excreted along with the oil. Olive and other vegetable oils can be substituted.

Foods Highest in Vitamin D. These include fish-liver oils, eggs, vitamin D fortified milk and milk products, bone meal, organ meats, fish (especially cod, herring, tuna, sardines, and salmon).

VITAMIN E

The minimum daily requirement for fat-soluble vitamin E has not been established, but the vitamin E requirement is unusually high for men during their reproductive years, for women after menopause, and for all obese people. Vitamin E is sold as mixed tocopherols or as d-alpha tocopherols. Research indicates that only the alpha tocopherol can function as a vitamin. Vitamin E is never toxic, but people who have had rheumatic heart disease or who have high blood pressure should begin with a low dosage of 90 I.U. a day for 1 month, and then 120 I.U. for the second month, and 150 I.U. for the third month, etc., until adequate therapeutic levels are reached. If reactions are unfavorable at any point, the level should be maintained at the amount just before the reaction. If a dosage of 400 I.U. or more is used by someone with a weak heart without preparation, it can strengthen the tone of the heart muscle so dramatically that it can cause the blood pressure to shoot up to dangerous levels.

Vitamin E serves as an antioxidant. Unless there is adequate vitamin E in the body, several nutrients are destroyed when they are exposed to oxygen coming into the body, including essential fatty acids (vitamin F, present in vegetable oils), carotene (a form of vitamin A), vitamin A, B vitamins (indirectly), and the pituitary, adrenal, and sex hormones. Vitamin E is necessary for normal reproduction and helps to prevent sterility and miscarriages. It prevents calcium deposits in blood vessel walls and is valuable in treatment of heart conditions and cardio-vascular diseases because it strengthens capillary walls and thus decreases clotting. It also reduces the body's need for oxygen and acts as a regulator of the metabolism of the cell nucleus. Vitamin E helps prevent or remove scars. A lack of vitamin E may cause a loss of reproductive powers, muscular disorders, nervousness and general weakness, impairment of iron absorption and hemoglobin formation so that red blood cells become fragile. A deficiency also results in the destruction of essential fatty acids by oxygen, and since these acids are part of the cell structure, this can result in clotting disorders.

The more oil or fat you eat, the more vitamin E you need. This vitamin is also destroyed by taking iron salts within 12 hours of taking vitamin E. It is also destroyed by radiation and X-rays. For the best absorption of vitamin E, vitamin C should be present.

Foods Highest in Vitamin E. These include raw wheat germ oil, whole-grain breads and cereals, margarine, eggs, and organ meats. Breast milk from a healthy mother contains about 20 times as much vitamin E as cow's milk. *Note*: 90 percent of the vitamin E in oils is destroyed by cooking.

IRON

Minimum Daily Requirements: Pregnant and Lactating Women: 20 mg.
Women, Boys, Girls: 15 mg.
Men, Children under 11: 10 mg.

Iron is needed by the body to make hemoglobin, which is the component in red blood that carries oxygen to each cell; oxygen is required for all bodily processes, particularly the production of energy. A lack of iron may result in constant fatigue and lack of endurance, pale complexion, shortness of breath, dizziness, headaches, and mental depression.

Magnesium, vitamin B6, and vitamin C all need to be present for the best absorption of iron.

Foods Highest in Iron (over 5 mg.). These include organ meats, clams, oysters, dulse seaweed (2/3 teaspoon), kelp (1 teaspoon), Irish moss or agar seaweed (1/4 cup), red kidney beans, soybeans, steamed dandelion greens, dried or canned apricots, prune juice, rice polish (1/3 cup), wheat germ (1 cup), sesame seeds (1/2 cup; raw seeds won't digest unless you're a religious chewer, so buy them roasted or roast them in a 350° oven for about 15 minutes, shaking the pan every few minutes, until golden brown—or grind them), brewer's yeast (3 tablespoons), blood (the best source of iron).

CALCIUM

Minimum Daily Requirements Boys: 1400 mg.
                                       Girls, Pregnant and Lactating Women:
                                        1300 mg.
                                        Men, Children under 11: 800 mg.

Calcium builds and maintains bones and teeth, helps blood to clot, aids vitality and endurance, regulates heart rhythm, and maintains muscle tone. A lack of calcium may result in tension, nervousness, headaches, insomnia, mental depression, water retention, low resistance to infections, and muscle cramps. (Note that all of these symptoms have been associated with menstrual problems; about 10 days before the period begins, the blood calcium level drops).

When calcium is taken in excessively large amounts, too much magnesium is excreted, resulting in kidney stones or diarrhea (which happens with some bottle-fed babies and ulcer patients). Phosphorus is also lost. Calcium may be deposited in joints and/or veins.

For the best absorption of calcium, you need about half as much magnesium as calcium. If you get more magnesium than that, it will deplete the calcium level. You also need protein, B vitamins, vitamin C, and vitamin D.

Foods Highest in Calcium (over 300 mg.). These include the following steamed greens: collard, mustard, turnip, dandelion, lamb's quarters. Also high in calcium are milk (1 cup), cheddar cheese, Swiss cheese, sardines, kelp (2 tablespoons), Irish moss or agar seaweed (3 tablespoons), sesame seeds (1/3 cup; raw seeds won't digest unless you're a religious chewer, so buy them roasted or roast them in a 350° oven for about 15 minutes, shaking the pan every few minutes, until golden brown—or grind them), calcium-fortified torula yeast (2 tablespoons), and bone meal or powder. *Note*: Oxalic acid released while cooking spinach, beet greens, dock, and sorrel interfere with calcium and possibly iron absorption. Calcium absorption is also impaired by eating chocolate.

MAGNESIUM

Minimum Daily Requirements: Pregnant and Lactating Women: 450 mg.
Men, Women, Boys, Girls: 350 mg.
Children under 11: 200 mg.

Magnesium maintains the normal functioning of the brain, spinal cord, and all nerves. A lack of magnesium may result in diarrhea; tremors; muscle spasms of the arms, hands, legs, feet, and eyes, or epileptic-like convulsions; and psychosis. Excessive intake of magnesium will result in the hoarding of the available albumin, crowding out the calcium and causing it to be lost in the urine.

Magnesium is lost rapidly when drinking alcohol or eating refined foods, sugar, and hydrogenated fats. For the best absorption of magnesium, you should also have protein and calcium (calcium intake should be about double that of magnesium).

Foods Highest in Magnesium (over 100 mg.). These include soy flour (1/3 cup), whole wheat flour (1 cup), raisin bran (1 cup), wheat bran (1 1/2 tablespoons), wheat germ (5 tablespoons), blackstrap molasses (2 tablespoons), kelp (1 tablespoon), almonds (1/4 cup), Brazil nuts (2 1/2 tablespoons), cashews (1/2 cup), peanuts (1/4 cup), dry sesame seeds (1/4 cup, raw seeds won't digest unless you're a religious chewer, so buy them roasted or roast them in a 350° oven for about 15 minutes, shaking the pan every few minutes, until golden brown—or grind them), steamed Swiss chard (1 cup), and steamed collard greens (1 cup). The diet of the average adult contains only about half of the daily requirements of this mineral.

Food grown in soil treated with lime or with chemical fertilizers containing potassium do not have much magnesium or trace elements. If you have a garden, try using dolomite instead of lime, and compost or organic fertilizers instead of chemical fertilizers.

Resources

All of the remedies listed in this book are readily available, though you may have to look beyond the familar drug store. Health food stores, herbal pharmacies, oriental pharmacies, and food co-ops are usually the best sources of herbal products. Even if there is no such store nearby, there are many mail-order businesses that carry these products. Here is a partial listing of places you can contact for a mail-order catalog listing various herbal, homeopathic, and naturopathic remedies. Some of these companies are mentioned in the text.

Ellon Bach, USA, Inc.
P.O. Box 320 Woodmere, NY 11598
(Bach flower remedies)

Bach (Canada)
Box 68, Station J
Toronto, Ontario M4J 4X8
Canada
(Bach flower remedies)

Battle Creek Equipment Company
307 West Jackson Street
Battle Creek, Michigan 49016
(Thermophores)

Bioforce of America Ltd.
21 West Mall
Plainview, NY 11808
(Bioforce Pollinosan)

Folklore Herbs
2388 W. 4th Ave.
Vancouver, B.C. V7K 1P1
Canada

The Herb Room
1130 Mission
Santa Cruz, CA 95060

Herbal Holding Company
P.O. Box 5854-W
Sherman Oaks, CA 91413
(Tibetan eye charts)

Indiana Botanic Gardens
PO Box 5
Hammond, IN 46325

Nature's Herbs
281 Ellis Street
San Francisco, CA 94102

Penn Herb Company
603 North 2nd Street
Philadelphia, PA 19123

San Francisco Herb and Natural Food Company
4543 Horton Steet
Emeryville, CA 94608

Standard Homeopathic Company
Box 61067
Los Angeles, California 90061
(Homeopathic preparations)

References

Aihara, Herman, *Acid and Alkaline* (Onoville, Calif.: The George Ohsawa Macrobiotic Foundation, 1971).

Airola, Paavo, N.D., *How to Get Well* (Phoenix, Ariz.: Health Plus, 1974).

Beard, Toni Roberts, et al, *Healthwise Handbook* (Boise, Idaho, 1976).

Biehler, Henry G., *Food Is Your Best Medicine* (New York: Vintage Books, 1973).

Boston Women's Health Book Collective, *Our Bodies Ourselves—A Book By and For Women* (New York: Simon & Schuster, 1971).

Botwinick, Jack, Ph.D., *Aging and Behavior* (New York: Springer Publishing Co., 1973).

Bricklin, Mark, *The Practical Encyclopedia of Natural Healing* (Emmaus, Pa.: Rodale Books, Inc. 1976).

Clark, Linda, *The Best of Linda Clark* (New Canaan, Conn.: Keats Publishing, Inc., 1976).

Davis, Adelle, *Let's Get Well* (New York: Harcourt, Brace and World, 1965).

Davis, Adelle, *Let's Have Healthy Children* (New York: Signet, 1972).

DeGowin, Elmer L., M.D., and DeGowin, Richard L., M.D., *Bedside Diagnostic Examination*, 3rd ed. (New York: MacMillan Publishing Co., 1976).

Ensminger, Ensminger, Konlade, and Robson, *Foods and Nutrition Encyclopedia* (Clovis, Calif., 1983).

An Explanatory Book of the Newest Illustration of Acupuncture Points (Hong Kong: Medicine and Health Publishing Co., 1973).

Ford Heritage, *Composition and Facts About Food* (Mokelumne Hill, Calif.: Health Research, 1971).

Grieve, Mrs. Maude, *A Modern Herbal* (New York: Dover Publications, 1971).

Hay, Louise L., *Heal Your Body, The Mental Causes for Physical Illness and the Metaphysical Way to Overcome Them* (Santa Monica, Calif: Hay House, 1988).

Horwitz, Nathan, "Breast Baby's Colic Linked to Mother's Drink of Cow's Milk," *Medical Tribune*, December 6, 1978.

Howell, Mary, M.D., *Healing at Home* (Boston: Beacon Press, 1978).

Jarvis, D.C., M.D., *Folk Medicine* (Greenwich, Conn.: Fawcett Crest, 1958).

Kalokerinos, Archie, *Every Second Child* (Australia: Thomas Nelson Limited, distributed by the Wholesale Nutrition Club, Sunnyvale, Calif., 1974)

Kirschmann, John D., *Nutrition Almanac* (New York: McGraw-Hill, 1975).

Kloss, Jethro, *Back to Eden* (Coalmont, Tenn.: Langview Publishing House, 1970).

Lerch, Constance, *Maternity Nursing* (St. Louis: The C.V. Mosby Co., 1972).

Lust, John, N.D., *The Herb Book* (New York: Bantam Books, 1974).

Marriott, Philip J., "Staphylococcal Skin Disease," *Nursing Times*, June 24, 1976.

Martindale, *The Extra Pharmacopoeia*, 26th ed., Normal W. Blacow, ed. (London: The Pharmaceutical Press, 1972).

The Medical Letter, Vol. 19, No. 4, February 25, 1977.

Mogabgag, William, and Pollack, Beatrice, "Re: Increased Virus Shedding with Aspirin Treatment of Rhino-virus Infection," *Journal of the American Medical Association*, 235, 1976.

Nahmias, Andre J., "The Torch Complex," *Hospital Practice*, Vol. 9, No. 5, May, 1974.

Orkin, Milton, M.D., et al, *Scabies and Pediculosis* (Philadelphia: J.B. Lippincott, Co., 1972).

Parker, D.J., "Herpes Simplex of the Genitals," *Nursing Times*, Dec. 11, 1975.

Peat, Ray, *Nutrition for Women* (Eugene, Ore.: Blake College, 1975).

Pfeiffer, Carl, *Mental and Elemental Nutrients, A Physician's Guide to Nutrition and Health Care* (New Canaan, Conn.: Keats Publishing Co., 1975.

Reuben, David R., M.D., *Reader's Digest*, November, 1974.

Rinehart, J.F., and Mettier, S.R., "The Heart Valves and Muscle in Experimental Scurvy with Superimposed Infection. With Notes on the Similarity of the Lesion to Those of Rheumatic Fever," *American Journal of Pathology*, Vol. X, 1934.

Robenburg, Gerald N., *Compendium of Pharmaceuticals and Specialties*, 13th ed. (Toronto: Canadian Pharmaceutical Association, 1978).

Robertson, Laurel, et al, *Laurel's Kitchen: A Handbook for Vegetarian Cookery and Nutrition* (Berkeley, Calif.: Nilgiri Press, 1977).

Rock, Arthur, M.D., et al, *Textbook of Dermatology*, 3rd ed. (Oxford: Blackwell Scientific Publications, 1979).

Rodale, J.I. and staff, *The Complete Book of Vitamins*, (Emmaus, Pa.: Rodale Books, Inc., 1968).

Rosenberg, Harold, M.D., and Feldsmen, A.N., Ph.D., *The Doctor's Book of Vitamin Therapy, Megavitamins for Health* (New York: G.P. Putnam's Sons, 1974).

Ryan, Kenneth J., M.D., and Gibson, Don C., *Menopause and Aging, Summary Report and Selected Papers* (U.S. Department of Health, Education, and Welfare, 1971).

Shute, Wilfrid E., M.D. and Taub, Harold, J., *Vitamin E for Ailing and Healthy Hearts* (New York: Pyramid Books, 1975).

Stanley, Dr., "Increased Virus Shedding with Asprin Treatment of Rhinovirus Infection," *Journal of the American Medical Association*, 231, 1975.

Stimson, A.M, et al, United States Public Health Service, "Notes on Experimental Rheumatic Fever," *Public Health Reports*, 49, Volume 1, March 16, 1934.

Stone, Irwin, *The Healing Factor: Vitamin C Against Disease* (New York: Grosset and Dunlap, 1972).

Vickery, Donald M., M.D., and Fries, James F., M.D., *Take Care of Yourself, A Consumer's Guide to Medical Care* (Reading, Mass.: Addison-Wesley Publishing Co., 1976).

Watson, Jeanette E., R.N., *Medical-Surgical Nursing* (Philadelphia: W.B. Saunders Co., 1972).

Weiss, Kay, "What Medical Students Learn About Women," *Off Our Backs*, April-May 1975.

Werner, David, *Where There Is No Doctor: A Village Health Care Handbook* (Palo Alto, Calif.: The Hesperian Foundation, 1978).

Index

Ailments appear in **bold** type.